Bottle Service

Bottle Service

EDUCATION AND
ENCOURAGEMENT
FOR GUILT-FREE AND
SUCCESSFUL
FORMULA FEEDING

Mallory Whitmore

SIMON ELEMENT
New York Amsterdam/Antwerp London
Toronto Sydney/Melbourne New Delhi

SIMON
ELEMENT

An Imprint of Simon & Schuster, LLC
1230 Avenue of the Americas
New York, NY 10020

This publication contains the opinions and ideas of its author. It is intended to provide helpful and informative material on the subjects addressed in the publication. It is sold with the understanding that the author and publisher are not engaged in rendering medical, health, or any other kind of personal professional services in the book. The reader should consult his or her medical, health, or other competent professional before adopting any of the suggestions in this book or drawing inferences from it.

The author and publisher specifically disclaim all responsibility for any liability, loss, or risk, personal or otherwise, that is incurred as a consequence, directly or indirectly, of the use and application of any of the contents of this book.

First Simon Element trade paperback edition February 2026

SIMON ELEMENT is a registered trademark of Simon & Schuster, LLC

Simon & Schuster strongly believes in freedom of expression and stands against censorship in all its forms. For more information, visit BooksBelong.com.

For information about special discounts for bulk purchases, please contact Simon & Schuster Special Sales at 1-866-506-1949 or business@simonandschuster.com.

The Simon & Schuster Speakers Bureau can bring authors to your live event. For more information or to book an event, contact the Simon & Schuster Speakers Bureau at 1-866-248-3049 or visit our website at www.simonspeakers.com.

INTERIOR DESIGN BY KARLA SCHWEER

Manufactured in the United States of America

10 9 8 7 6 5 4 3 2 1

Library of Congress Control Number: 2025939104

ISBN 978-1-6680-8876-0 (pbk)
ISBN 978-1-6680-8877-7 (ebook)

*To my family, who inspires everything
I do and gives me the courage to do it*

Contents

Bottle Service

INTRODUCTION

Mom Note

I See You, Because I've Been There

My oldest daughter is almost ten. She is creative and kind, smart and silly, funny and hardworking, and so beautiful it hurts. She and her brother are two of the very best things to ever happen to me. And when she was born, I was convinced I had made the biggest mistake of my life.

Maybe your experience is different—perhaps you feel nothing but overwhelming love and gratitude for the little human in your arms. I am so thrilled for you! Truly. That just wasn't the case for me.

From the moment she arrived, I felt overwhelmed. Underwater. Totally and completely unprepared for the reality of having a tiny baby who was dependent on me for every one of her needs, night and day, relentlessly (or so it felt, even with a supportive partner). And you might be thinking, *Mallory, didn't you take any of those baby classes? Didn't you read any books?* The answer is yes. I took the classes. I read the books. I researched and learned and listened to experts and dug in deep on how to do this parenting thing "the right way."

And then my baby came along and the whole plan went to shit.

Because babies do that, right? They don't care about how they "should" behave, or what your goals are, or what the parenting books say. They only know how to cry and eat and poop, and frankly, they don't even do those last two very well at first. Babies are whole (albeit squishy) humans who come with their own set of needs and challenges that, unfortunately, can't be fully explored until they arrive earth-side.

The biggest source of my stress in those early days and weeks with my girl was trying to feed her. She was late preterm and wasn't motivated to eat. My milk was delayed due to a scheduled C-section and undiagnosed gestational diabetes. My daughter lost a lot of weight. I couldn't express any milk— not even drops—for days. Nurses and lactation consultants constantly manhandled me while my baby screamed, and often we both ended up crying, staring at my breasts, and wondering what to do next.

The nurses in the hospital started her on formula before we were discharged, due to the amount of weight she had lost, and I felt like the world's biggest failure. Like I had screwed her up for life by not being able to breastfeed her like everyone said I should. *Did I even want to breastfeed?* I'm not sure where the pressure began and any desire I had ended. *Did it even matter whether I wanted to breastfeed?* It certainly didn't feel like it. Instead, breastfeeding was positioned as the obvious choice for mothers who wanted the best for their babies—and who

wouldn't want that? Never mind the unspoken message behind this narrative: *Not* breastfeeding means you didn't care
enough—or didn't try hard enough—to give your baby the
best.

So I tried harder. My milk came in, and I started pumping. (To this day, the rhythmic whirring of a breast pump
makes my heart rate increase and my cortisol spike.) We
kept giving our daughter formula and whatever milk I could
produce, and she started gaining weight. She began doing
a lot better, but my mental health got a lot worse. The
relentlessness of pumping around the clock and *still* not
being able to meet her needs made me feel useless; I was
working so hard to feed her and still coming up short day
after day. I hated being stuck next to an outlet, having the
milk (and the life, it felt like) sucked out of me eight to
twelve times a day and it never being enough. I felt like *I*
wasn't enough.

After an intervention from my sister, another from my
husband, and two grace-filled conversations with my doctor
and my daughter's pediatrician, we switched to exclusively
formula feeding when our daughter was six weeks old. It ended
one of the toughest seasons of my life—the one where I tried,
unsuccessfully, to breastfeed.

This decision came with a lot of emotions. I felt free, and
I felt guilty for feeling free. I felt relieved, and then I felt
ashamed because I felt relieved. I felt grateful for formula
and scared someone would see me with it in my shopping
cart. But mostly? Mostly, I felt confused.

I had done all the hard work to learn about breastfeeding!

I took the hospital's class, worked with lactation consultants, owned the books, and talked with friends and family who had done it successfully! The problem, at that point, was I knew basically nothing about formula or formula feeding.

Unmoored by this, I set out to become the best formula feeder I could be. I started scouring the internet for resources or support groups or books but found pretty much nothing. In 2016, the information about formula on the internet was limited to manufacturer websites and thinly veiled breastfeeding support pages with formula sections that said, in prettier language, "Don't do it."

How could there be thousands of experts on Instagram, weekly clinics at the hospital, dozens of subreddits, and tons of books about breastfeeding, yet basically nothing for formula feeding? Especially when the CDC (as I'd soon learn) reports that 75 percent of US families are *not* exclusively breastfeeding by the time their baby is six months old?

So many of us are using formula, I thought—*certainly I can't be the only one who doesn't know what I'm doing and who also feels really guilty about it.* A seed of an idea started then—to create the type of community I needed in that moment—but I didn't have the capacity to nurture the seed as an overwhelmed new mom. Instead, I struggled through my daughter's first year feeling isolated and wondering, constantly, if I was doing right by her. It wasn't the first year of parenting I wanted to have, and so much of the difficulty was a result of our feeding journey.

When our son was born almost three years later, my husband and I made the decision to use formula from day one.

This was the absolute best decision for us (and one I've never regretted for a second)! *There must be better information out there this time*, I thought—and there still wasn't. It was then, early in the COVID pandemic with a toddler and a baby, that I decided to launch an Instagram page, which eventually turned into a profitable business called The Formula Mom. I wanted to offer the sort of support and information I was desperate for and still couldn't find.

I tell you this story for two reasons:

First, because I want you to know *I've been where you are*. I don't know the details of your story, your pregnancy or birth, or your feeding journey. Your path to formula might look completely different from either of my experiences, and that's fine! That's not what matters. What matters is that you know whatever you're feeling about your baby's feeding experience—overwhelm, grief, relief, frustration, annoyance, sadness, or hope—I've felt it, too. I'm convinced no one escapes the first year of feeding a baby without feeling a full spectrum of emotions. I've been where you are, even if our situations aren't identical.

And second, I want you to know *you can end up where I am*. It is possible for you to feel confident while feeding your baby with formula. It's possible to have joy when you think back on your baby's feeding journey. It's possible to reframe what you might consider failure now and view it as success down the line. Perhaps most pressingly at this point in your baby's first year, I want you to know that feeding your baby doesn't have to feel quite so isolating and hard.

I've become an expert over the years (more on this in the next chapter!), but I'm a parent first.

This book is a love letter to Mallory in 2016, who was scared she didn't have what it took to be a great mom. And it's also my love letter to you, with all my hope it'll help you know you're already a great parent to your baby.

1

What to Expect from
Bottle Service

The last chapter covered my personal why behind this book; now we'll focus on the broader why, what, and how.

Why Formula Education Matters

The reality is that only about one-fourth of US families are exclusively breastfeeding at their baby's half birthday, meaning that a large number of families are feeding formula. And yet so few receive any formal guidance about how to do so safely and successfully. In a 2023 survey conducted on behalf of Willow, Bobbie, and SimpliFed, nearly 50 percent of mothers reported receiving "little to no support/education around formula feeding." In 2024, the Centers for Disease Control and Prevention (CDC) shared information about a longitudinal study that found that out of four thousand women surveyed, only 12 percent of parent respondents reported being instructed by a health care provider on how to prepare formula.

With an approach similar to abstinence-only sex education, the prevailing belief is that educating about formula or sharing ways formula can benefit parents will encourage more to formula feed. *But most American parents are formula feeding already*. According to moms, withholding formula education wouldn't change how long they would breastfeed. Instead, it aids in decreasing parental competence and confidence about how to use formula. This is a cost parents—and infants—shouldn't have to bear.

While parents need fundamental formula education, they also need encouragement and support. In the same brand survey, fewer than 25 percent of parents reported feeling proud about using formula to feed their babies (compared to more than 70 percent of breastfeeding parents who took pride in their feeding choice). While most mothers (65 percent) reported feeling judged for their feeding decisions, mothers who were exclusively formula feeding reported the *most* judgment. In a 2021 Wakefield study that looked at the impact of infant feeding choices on mental health, nearly half of respondents indicated that at least one feeding-related challenge had hurt their mental health, with more than a quarter admitting that challenges with breastfeeding had a negative impact.

In a "breast is best" world where nursing is seen as a moral issue (and formula feeding as a moral failure), parents using formula are often left to navigate their lack of knowledge and negative feelings alone.

It's time to change the narrative, don't you think?

All parents deserve to feel confident, successful, and joyful during their infant's feeding journey regardless of what, or how, they feed their baby. If this is what you are after, you're in the right place.

How to Read *Bottle Service*

Bottle Service is a reference guide to help parents and caregivers understand the art and science of bottle feeding and its related challenges. The book *does not* need to be read chronologically from beginning to end; it is organized in two different ways to make it easier for tired new parents to find the information they need.

First, the book is structured by baby age. Each section covers an age range and includes topics that parents commonly have questions about during the indicated months. Second, the book contains three types of content: educational chapters, actionable pieces of advice (known as Quick Tips), and supportive vignettes (called Mom Notes). There is also a comprehensive index at the back that directs to specific topics at their respective page numbers. Feel free to skip around to whatever information you need when you need it!

What You'll Find Inside

While you will find summary information provided, with references, by the American Academy of Pediatrics (AAP) and other medical organizations, *this book is intended for educational purposes only and is not medical advice.* I am not a physician, and more importantly, I am not your child's physician! Please review any strategies or suggestions from this book with your child's pediatrician before implementing, as they (and you!) know your baby best.

Additionally, the strategies laid out in this book are intended for healthy, full-term infants and may not be appropriate for babies born prematurely or for those with medical diagnoses. If you are unsure whether the information contained herein is appropriate for your infant, please discuss this content with their pediatrician or care team.

Finally, the information provided is based on US guidelines and recommendations, and may not align with guidelines from other regulatory and advisory bodies, including those in Canada and Europe. Given this, readers from outside the US should defer to the guidelines and recommendations given by their applicable regulatory bodies.

My goal—as a parent and an educator—is to present quality research and best practices in a way that is easy for parents to digest. I aggregate information from a variety of sources, including but not limited to the AAP, the World Health Organization (WHO), US Food and Drug Administration (FDA), CDC, a variety of peer-reviewed journals, and expert interviews. All relevant sources are cited with trailing phrase endnotes in the back matter of this book.

A Note About Language

I am a mother of two, and my business name references how I self-identify: The Formula Mom. I recognize, however, that not all formula feeding parents are women, not all families include a mother, and that there are a variety of ways a reader of this book may identify outside of the "male" and "female" and/or "mother" and "father" binaries.

I believe one of the best and biggest benefits of bottle feeding is that anyone can feed a baby successfully, regardless of their anatomy, identity, or relationship to the infant. As such, I use *mom*, *parent*, and *caregiver* interchangeably in this book. As mothers historically take on the bulk of feeding duties, I rely on this identifier more heavily than others. This is not meant to be exclusionary but instead meant to reflect the reality of most infant feeding relationships. Please view all content through the lens most appropriate to you and your infant, regardless of how the caregiver relationship is described on the page.

Additionally, I refer to the act of nursing as *breastfeeding* for ease of comprehension. I acknowledge that some parents or caregivers prefer the term *chestfeeding* or *bodyfeeding* and that any of these terms can refer to feeding expressed milk in addition to, or instead of, feeding from the body. I refer to the output of nursing or pumping as *breast milk* or *human milk*. These terms are meant to mirror the language used most commonly by medical associations and society at large. Please view all content through the lens most appropriate to you and your infant, regardless of how the body, or the function of producing milk, is described on the page.

2

What Is Baby Formula?

People have *a lot* of opinions about what formula is (and isn't). A few you might have heard: Formula is poison, formula isn't as good as breast milk, formula is industrially processed food, formula is a man-made product for selfish parents. These all describe *beliefs* about infant formula, but none capture the essential question: What is formula made of, and why? To answer this, we must start from the beginning—because contrary to popular belief, there has never been a time when all mothers breastfed.

A Brief History of Infant Formula Across Time

Lactation failure, or the inability to successfully breastfeed, was first noted in an Egyptian publication, the Papyrus Ebers, from 1550 BCE. It included a recommendation to induce lactation and/or increase milk supply by rubbing the oily bones of a swordfish on a woman's back, which has since fallen out of favor—obviously. This provided the first written evidence that breastfeeding has *always* been a challenge for some parents. In these cases, wet-nursing was long the primary method of alternative feeding when direct nursing wasn't available (or, in the case of women with higher status, wasn't desired). This lasted for millennia, until the early nineteenth century, when "artificial feeding became a feasible substitute for wet nursing."

Even with the prevalence of wet-nursing throughout history, there has always been evidence of artificial feeding—feeding babies substances other than human milk—as demonstrated by the discovery of "clay feeding vessels" in newborn burial sites from as early as 2000 BCE. These vessels were confirmed to be used for infant feeding after analysis of residues found within showed casein proteins, a key feature of animal milk. By the sixteenth century, some infants were fed animal milk along with a mixture known as "pap" or "panada," which was made using a grain product like bread or cereal soaked in water, broth, or milk.

The first commercial infant formula was developed around 1865 by Justus von Liebig, a German chemist who combined cow's milk, potassium bicarbonate, malt flour, and wheat flour into a product he marketed as the first infant food. From there, innovation boomed, leading to patents for twenty-seven different brands of infant foods by 1883. By 1929, a Committee on Foods was formed by the American Medical Association to oversee the safety and quality of infant formula and issue a "seal of acceptance" for approved products. This was a precursor to the work now done by the US Food and Drug Administration (FDA).

Several decades later, the United States Congress passed the Infant Formula Act of 1980, which established "minimum nutrient requirements, define[d] adulteration, and provide[d] for establishing nutrient and quality control procedures, prescribe[d] recall procedures, and specifie[d] inspection requirements." These requirements are still enforced by the FDA today, though certain provisions have been updated over the intervening years as the understanding of infant nutrition science and food safety has evolved.

Formula Composition Today

Infant formula, by design, is a breast milk substitute. It is a product that can be used alongside or in place of human milk to provide complete nutrition for infants zero through twelve months. To create infant formulas, scientists and manufacturers isolate, process, and combine a variety of ingredients and nutrients—such as milk, lactose, and plant-based oils—to provide a nutrient profile that is clinically shown to support healthy infant growth and development.

That's right! *Every infant formula that is legally sold in the US must meet FDA regulatory requirements to demonstrate that the formula is both safe and nutritionally adequate for infants.* In fact, infant formula is one of the most highly regulated foods you can buy. These regulations are important due to the vulnerable nature of new babies and the critical developmental period of the first year of life.

The most frequent question parents have for me when considering using formula? They want to know how formula compares to breast milk nutritionally. When considering macronutrients (fat, carbs, and protein—more on this in chapter 5!) and micronutrients (vitamins and minerals), formula composition is crafted to be similar to what is found in breast milk. This is because formula is specifically designed to be an effective substitute for infant feeding, so every effort is made to model the nutrient composition of breast milk as closely as possible!

There are some features of breast milk, however, like bioactive components, that formula cannot currently replicate. These components include hormones, antibodies, stem cells, and growth factors, among others. These properties change in type and volume over time, as breast milk evolves to meet babies' changing needs as they age. While infant formulas do not contain these properties, the nutritive content of infant formula is designed to be very similar to breast milk.

"But don't babies need bioactive components, like antibodies from breast milk, to stay healthy? Are formula-fed babies sicker because they don't receive these?"

Antibodies are proteins that the body's immune system makes to destroy harmful substances called *antigens*. Maternal antibodies, passed through the placenta and/or through breast milk, provide the baby with a type of immunity called *passive immunity*. This type of immunity differs from *active immunity*, or the kind that occurs as a result of a prior infection or in response to a vaccine. While both types of immunity lay an important foundation for health, they differ in their duration of benefit. Passive immunity provides the advantage of offering immediate benefit; however, these immediate benefits are thought to only last a few weeks or months. Maternal antibodies passed through breast milk are protective against certain disease-carrying organisms.

It's also worth noting that, even though some studies demonstrate a reduction in respiratory, ear, and gastrointestinal infections in breastfed infants compared to formula-fed infants, other factors like pacifier use and group childcare also influence the odds an infant will get sick in their first year of life. It's important to remember that the immune system is complex and is developed over time by many factors, both inside and outside of a parent's control. How you feed your baby is just one variable of many that influence their response to pathogens.

Types of Formulas

There are several different categories of formula on the market, though all infant formulas intended for healthy, full-term babies provide roughly equivalent nutrition (remember, they have to meet the same regulatory guidelines!). I like to categorize infant formulas based on protein size—which affects digestibility—and how they are marketed based on digestive symptom(s). Here's a primer:

Routine or Standard: These formulas tend to be the starting point for most feeding journeys. They typically include cow's milk or goat's milk as a base and feature intact milk proteins, lactose as the carbohydrate source (lactose is a naturally occurring sugar found in mammal milks like cow's milk and breast milk), and a blend of plant-based oils in addition to vitamins and minerals. Intact milk proteins mean that the protein is complete and not broken down in any way, and an article published by the AAP suggests that most infants do well on this type of formula.

Gentle: Also known as *tolerance formulas*, gentle formulas contain partially hydrolyzed, or broken down, milk proteins. Breaking up the protein into smaller pieces is marketed to be easier to digest, with the AAP suggesting that these types of proteins may address crying, fussiness, colic symptoms, and gas. Often, gentle formulas include a carbohydrate blend, including lactose along with an alternative like corn syrup, glucose syrup, maltodextrin, or sucrose. Some gentle formulas include no lactose at all.

Sensitive: In my opinion, "sensitive" is a bit of a misnomer, as these formulas contain the same intact protein that we see in routine formulas. They also tend to include less whey protein than a routine formula, which can make them *harder* to digest, not easier! The key feature of a sensitive formula is intact milk protein and very little (if any) lactose for carbohydrates. Instead, most use corn syrup or maltodextrin. These formulas are typically marketed for gas and fussiness.

Hypoallergenic: Also known as *HA* formulas, hypoallergenic formulas are a group that include extensively hydrolyzed (broken down) milk protein-based formulas and free amino acid–based formulas.

Extensively Hydrolyzed Formulas: In a hypoallergenic formula, the proteins are broken down to such an extent that at least 90 percent of infants with clinically documented cow's milk allergies will not react to them. Nearly all are lactose-free, making them a common recommendation for infants with galactosemia— a rare congenital enzyme deficiency. Some also contain MCT oil in place of or in addition to more common plant-based oils to allow for easier fat absorption. These formulas are intended for infants with cow milk protein allergy or intolerance (CMPA/CMPI), milk soy protein intolerance (MSPI), and other medical needs. Outside of these diagnoses, extensively hydrolyzed formulas are often marketed for treatment of colic and reflux.

Amino Acid or Elemental Formulas: Amino acid formulas, also known as *elemental formulas*, do not contain milk proteins at all. Instead, they contain the building blocks of protein—amino acids. These formulas are lactose-free and often contain MCT oil for easier fat absorption. Elemental formulas are recommended for the small portion of infants with one or more food allergies who react to extensively hydrolyzed formulas and/or those who have medical conditions that impact nutrient absorption (such as cystic fibrosis). Amino acid formulas are often the final commercially available formula option for infants who have not done well with—or who have struggled to gain appropriate weight on—other over-the-counter formulas. For infants who cannot tolerate an amino acid–based formula, specialized medical formulas are available by prescription from medical retailers.

Specialty: There are a few formula types that fall outside of these buckets and therefore get lumped into a "specialty" category. These include soy formulas, formulas for premature babies, thickened formulas (sometimes called *added rice*, *AR*, or *anti-reflux* formulas), and metabolic and other medical formulas. It is recommended to consult with your child's doctor when selecting any infant formula, including before using a specialty formula, as there are criteria for use that should be considered.

Formula Formats

In addition to these categories based largely on protein size and ingredients, formulas come in three different formats: liquid concentrate, liquid ready-to-feed, and powder. Each offers a number of pros and cons.

Liquid concentrate formula is less popular than powder formula and has lost favor over the years. Concentrate formula comes in cans and must be mixed with water according to the label instructions before serving. While concentrate formula is sterile (a plus) and less expensive than liquid ready-to-feed, it can come with logistical challenges. The cans are heavy to carry around in a diaper bag and must be refrigerated after opening, making them challenging to use on the go. Additionally, formula concentrate is sometimes harder to find given its declining popularity.

Liquid ready-to-feed formula is the most convenient of the formats, as it lives up to its name—it's ready to feed to your baby without any dilution! Simply pour into a bottle (or screw a nipple onto the top of preportioned two-ounce bottles available for sale) and you're good to go! Like liquid concentrate, ready-to-feed formulas are sterile, which makes them the recommended choice of many pediatricians for preemies and newborns who are more susceptible to illness. As the most expensive formula format based on price per fluid ounce, ready-to-feed formulas are not often used long-term, though they are—like all infant formulas—nutritionally complete for healthy, full-term infants ages zero to twelve months. Ready-to-feed formulas must also be refrigerated after opening.

Powdered formula is the most popular format, offering more affordability, accessibility, and variety than the liquid options. These formulas must be mixed with water according to the directions on the label before serving! Powdered formula is not sterile, and as such, some pediatricians and health authorities recommend waiting to introduce it until your baby reaches a certain age or milestone. Before you panic, remember that expressed breast milk is also not sterile; sterility isn't a requirement for safe infant feeding! Your pediatrician can advise on their recommended timeline for introducing powdered formula to your infant. Many parents find powdered formula to be convenient, as it is easy to preportion, it's available at many retailers in person and online, and it tends to be cheaper per fluid ounce compared to liquid varieties.

Formula Is...

Infant formula is a product made from a highly regulated combination of ingredients to provide crucial nutrients for infants as a supplement to or replacement for breast milk. But more than that, formula is food. Formula is comfort. Formula is the product of some of the best minds in human milk science and infant nutrition. Rest assured that the ingredients in your baby's formula are just a small part of what formula provides: sustenance, growth, chunky leg and arm rolls, and the opportunity to bond with your baby multiple times every day as you feed them. Formula is the vehicle for healthy development for the majority of babies you know, and it could be for your baby, too.

3

Bottle Feeding from Birth—Planning Ahead

Whether you intend to formula feed from day one or simply want to prepare for any possible outcome, it's wise to start thinking about feeding logistics before your baby arrives! You'll want to consider the research you should do during pregnancy, the items you'll want to bring to the hospital, and how you might prepare your home for feeding a baby. But before we get into those logistics, let's take a moment to talk about best-laid plans.

On Plans and Expectations

Expecting a baby is exciting . . . and can provoke anxiety. One particularly tricky part? *Making decisions while having incomplete information.* As expecting parents, we try our best to make calls (about what size onesies to start with, which diaper brand to choose, whether to get a bouncer or a swing, and more), but we can only do so without full context. Any decision made before a baby arrives is made without knowledge of certain variables. We don't yet know how we will react to new parenthood, what our needs will be, or what our baby's needs and preferences will look like. As such, any advice you receive before your baby is earth-side should be taken with a grain of salt—even my advice! Any plans you make should be held loosely.

Because here's the thing: It's easy to make decisions when they exist only in the context of a future ideal state where everything turns out the way you envision it. It's harder to execute on those decisions when you come up against obstacles or circumstances you hadn't accounted for previously. Every parent learns new information about themselves, and their baby, on the other side of their birth. This new information—about things you find painful, or the anatomy of your baby's mouth, or how you react to waking up every two hours each night for weeks on end—can and should impact your plans.

Repeat after me: Changing your mind when you have more information isn't failure, it's wisdom.

This is a frequent mantra of mine, even ten years into parenting!

It is not a failure to make a different choice than you intended once all the variables come into focus. Instead, it is wise to look critically at the circumstances that surround a decision and evaluate whether what you thought would be best—when you didn't know what you know now—still is.

Feeding a baby isn't like following a treasure map that has one single route to the chest of gold (a healthy, growing baby). Instead, it's a scavenger hunt; you pick up clues along the way and make adjustments about where you're heading based on what you've learned. Treating your feeding journey this way will result in a happier, more relaxed experience—I promise.

Interested but Wary About Formula? Check the Research!

"Interested but wary about formula" was my state of mind during my first pregnancy. Had I been honest with myself and others, I probably would have admitted I never felt a strong desire to breastfeed. But I planned for it and tried it anyway because I was under the impression my baby would be *so much better off* if I nursed her. This is the prevailing narrative that you are likely to hear, but it lacks context. Learning what high-quality research shows about formula versus breastfeeding outcomes can be helpful in making an informed decision about how you plan to feed. I recommend Emily Oster's book *Cribsheet* as a go-to source for evidence-based summaries of the research behind many fraught parenting decisions, including how you feed.

If You Are Intending to Formula Feed

We used formula from day one with our second child, and it was, without a doubt, the best decision for us. Nearly seven years later, I have never once—even for a second—

regretted this choice. There are a number of factors for why a family would want or have to use formula from the start, and the reasons matter very little. The plan is the same regardless!

If you want to prepare to use formula from day one, consider taking the following steps.

Before birth, you should:

- Research and select the formula you plan to use (instructions for this process in chapter 5). I recommend having two weeks' worth of formula on hand, anticipating that you will prepare twenty to thirty fluid ounces of formula a day during the first two weeks of life. Given that formula is nonreturnable and often nonrefundable (for safety), and you won't know how your baby will take to a particular formula before they try it, I don't suggest purchasing more than this to start.

- Research and select the bottles you plan to use. Babies who are exclusively bottle fed tend to accept whatever bottle you start them with. For full-term babies without a medical condition that affects feeding or oral motor skills, I suggest Dr. Brown's or Evenflo Feeding Balance + bottles, as these feature a gradually sloping nipple with a wide base that allows for good latch! The number of bottles you need will depend on how frequently you want to wash them. Brand-new babies eat every two to three hours around the clock, averaging eight to twelve feedings a day. Having six bottles on hand, at minimum, is ideal.

- Learn the basics of how to prepare a bottle safely (see chapter 7) and make a practice bottle! You don't want your first experience to be in the middle of the night, in the dark, when you're running on adrenaline and three hours of sleep.

- Ask for your hospital's (or birthing center's) formula policy. Some hospitals do not allow parents to bring or use their own formula in the hospital due to safety and liability concerns. Others will allow this with pediatrician approval. Some only allow liquid ready-to-feed formula, while others allow powdered formula. Some may ask you to sign a waiver stating you understand that "breastfeeding is best" before they provide formula (you can refuse to sign). Some may only provide formula if they have determined there is sufficient medical need (don't get me started on this). Being prepared for whatever you might encounter in the hospital, and tailoring your plans appropriately based on what you learn, can help reduce stress after delivery.

- Pack feeding items in your hospital bag. Plan to bring formula (whatever kind you prefer and your hospital allows), bottles and nipples, a bottle brush, and dish soap. I was shocked when my hospital could only provide body wash when I asked to wash my pump parts and bottles in my postpartum room! You may also want to bring pacifiers, as some Baby-Friendly® hospitals no longer provide them.

- Inform your friends, family, and care team about your decision to formula feed. Being proactive in this effort can reduce the mental and emotional energy required for this conversation after birth (when you're likely to have less energy). I suggest being direct, confident, and final: "We've made the informed choice to formula feed [based on factors we don't wish to discuss]. We appreciate your support of this decision." When speaking with your care team before and after birth, ask that the decision to formula feed be noted in your chart along with your request to decline lactation support, if desired.

- Identify someone in your circle as your advocate while at the hospital or birthing center. This person is in charge of running interference if you receive pushback from the care team or staff lactation consultant about choosing to use formula. In a perfect world, your wishes would be respected the first time with no further discussion. In the real world, it's good to have someone appointed to remind new providers after every shift change what your wishes are and that you appreciate their commitment to honoring them.

- Set up your home for bottle feeding. Check out the Quick Tip on setting up a feeding station for a list of good-to-have products to make your life easier!

If You Are Open to Formula Feeding in Case That's Where the Journey Takes You

Why should those who intend to breastfeed be prepared for formula feeding?

Because it's better to have something you don't need than to need something you don't have.

No one makes their best decisions while sleep deprived with a new baby (the amount of money I spent on Amazon at two o'clock in the morning in 2016 is a testament to this). Putting thought into what you might do if breastfeeding doesn't go according to plan *before* you're in a feeding crisis is smart. Here are your tasks:

- Research and purchase a formula you would be comfortable using if needed or desired. I suggest having one or two cans or containers on hand. You can store these in a cabinet, and if you never use them, donate them to your local women's shelter! If you decide to use them, having one or two ready to go will buy you time to get more while avoiding the everyone-is-crying-and-overwhelmed-at-9:00-p.m. formula run.

- Purchase a set of bottles. For full-term babies without a medical condition that affects feeding or oral motor skills, I suggest Dr. Brown's or Evenflo Feeding Balance + bottles, as these feature a gradually sloping nipple with a wide base that allows for good latch!

- Learn about paced bottle feeding (and see chapter 8 on position while feeding). This is a bottle feeding technique that more closely mirrors the experience of feeding at the breast and can be helpful to use for combo feeding babies who alternate between nursing and bottle feeding.

- Review how to make a bottle safely and correctly (see chapter 7).

Feeding Is a Process

No matter how you plan to feed your baby, you will likely experience bumps and detours along the way. This is normal! The best thing you can do is remember that no one is born an expert (you or your baby) and that learning as you go is the best path forward. Happy feeding!

4

Drying Up Your Milk
(Whenever You're Ready)

Did you know that in all likelihood, you will experience your milk coming in after delivery even if you don't put your baby to your breast and never actually breastfeed? This catches parents off guard! While putting your baby to the breast *does* encourage milk production (the removal of milk signals the body to produce more), stage two lactogenesis—the onset of milk secretion after birth—occurs as a result of hormonal changes after the delivery of the placenta, regardless of whether you plan to nurse. If you've already decided to formula feed, dealing with this reality can come with discomfort at best and risk of inflammation or infection (such as mastitis) at worst.

Methods for Drying Up Your Milk Supply

In decades past, mothers who did not want to breastfeed were given the option to take medication(s) to suppress lactation, including one called Parlodel (bromocriptine)—a dopamine agonist that suppressed prolactin, the hormone responsible for milk production. However, the drug stopped being used for this purpose in 1994 amid consumer pressure and a threat to repeal approval from the FDA due to risks such as stroke, seizure, and heart attack.

The controversy was such that a health advocacy group sued the FDA for allowing Parlodel to be sold for the purpose of lactation suppression—at the time, it was used by three to six hundred thousand women a year—when there were thirty-two reported fatalities from the drug between 1980 and 1994. After the mid-1990s, medications to suppress lactation in new mothers were not routinely offered, and today, there are no drugs currently approved for this purpose in the United States.

Without an approved medication to help dry up milk, we are left with a variety of comfort measures, old wives' tales, and the passage of time to stop the flow.

Try These Tips!

Breast milk production works on a supply and demand model: When milk is removed from the breast, it signals the body to make more. As such, the number one tip for drying up milk is to *not* express it. We want the body to get the memo that no one is drinking the milk, and therefore it doesn't need to keep producing it! This means not putting your baby to your breast, not using a breast pump (manual or electric), and avoiding nipple stimulation in any form. If you had been nursing or pumping previously, you may need to take a slow and steady approach by lessening milk removal over time, either by decreasing your feeding duration or increasing the interval between feeding sessions. If you stop removing milk altogether too quickly, you could be at a greater risk for clogged ducts, engorgement, or mastitis! If you find yourself with extreme discomfort due to engorgement (breasts that feel overly full), you can hand-express a bit of milk to reduce discomfort.

You may choose to wear "milk collectors" to catch milk that falls during a letdown, as this can help you stay dry and provide a bit of nutrition, if desired, for your little one. These are small plastic or silicone collection cups that fit around and under the nipple but do not provide any suction. This is ideal, as suction—from a pump—will encourage more milk removal (and thus, more production). Other tips include:

- **Wear a tight-fitting, supportive bra.** In years past, women would bind their breasts to help dry up their milk! This is no longer encouraged, but you can achieve a similar (and more comfortable) result by wearing a tight-fitting bra—like a sports bra—that holds your breasts in place and prevents nipple stimulation from movement.

- **Consider using cabbage.** Bear with me, as I know this sounds bizarre! While the mechanism for benefit is debated (is it a sulfur compound, or some anti-inflammatory property, or the fact they're often applied chilled?), cabbage leaves have been shown in some research studies to reduce breast pain, hardness, and engorgement in lactating women, although there is low certainty in the evidence. Some moms prefer to separate the leaves of a white cabbage and freeze them on a baking sheet, as the cold temperature can provide relief and the cup of a cabbage leaf naturally shapes to the breast! For those who do not want to stuff cabbage in their bra, a product like CaboCréme—which contains enzymes from cabbage—can be applied several times a day to provide relief, although research indicates this approach is no more effective than placebo.

- **Drink sage tea.** Sage, an herb, is believed to help reduce milk production, although no scientific studies evaluate its effect. To make sage tea, steep one to three grams (each gram is roughly one-quarter of a teaspoon) in one cup of hot water. Because excess sage intake can result in side effects such as nausea and dizziness, it's advised to only drink one cup per twelve-hour period.

- **Get minty.** Peppermint oil, when mixed in a carrier oil, can be applied directly onto your breasts to potentially reduce engorgement and limit milk production. While no clinical trials have been conducted to support its effectiveness, studies in mice (using menthol) show suppression of milk production. *Only use peppermint oil on your breasts if you have completely stopped nursing, as you don't want your baby to ingest it!* Peppermint essential oil should be diluted in a ratio of two drops per one teaspoon of carrier oil (such as coconut or jojoba) before being applied to skin.

- **Apply ice packs.** This may not help reduce your milk supply but can help reduce discomfort while your body winds down production. Applying a cold gel pack can help make the weaning process more comfortable.

- **Be cautious of Sudafed.** Pseudoephedrine, a component in many over-the-counter decongestants, is known to significantly reduce milk supply in lactating women. One study showed a nearly 25 percent reduction in milk supply within twenty-four hours of participants taking a single sixty milligram dose. However, medications containing pseudoephedrine can cause side effects, including increased blood pressure and heart rate, nausea, and headaches. These symptoms can also be signs of postpartum preeclampsia, and you don't want to have to guess whether you're having a medical emergency postpartum or simply experiencing side effects from the medication. If you want to try Sudafed for drying up your milk, please do so with your doctor's sign-off and supervision!

Seek Professional Help

If you're unsure how to dry up your milk supply safely or if you need support during the process, consider reaching out to an International Board Certified Lactation Consultant (IBCLC). They are experts in all things lactation! Be aware, though, that some may encourage you to keep breastfeeding. Finding a practitioner who is supportive of your wishes—and your desired feeding journey—will be important here. Your primary care physician can also be a good resource during this process.

Give It Time

No matter what strategies you use to help your body dry up its milk, be prepared for the process to take several weeks (or even longer if you have been nursing or pumping and need to wean slowly, dropping a feeding every five days or so). You may find that you still produce a small amount of milk months down the line if you attempt to hand-express! Weaning too fast can increase your chances of developing mastitis—a spectrum of conditions resulting from inflammation and edema. If you experience fever, a breast that's warm and red to the touch, and/or chills and body aches, check with your doctor about whether treatment for mastitis is needed.

No matter when you attempt to stop producing milk, it can be a slow and uncomfortable process. Being prepared for stage two lactogenesis after birth—and having some of the items above on hand—can help make the process easier!

BABY AGE

0-3 Months

5

Choosing a Baby Formula

Ask any parent what they want in a formula and nearly all of them will say they want "the closest one to breast milk." Fear not! All regulated infant formulas are good formulas, and all are modeled after breast milk to provide the macronutrients and micronutrients infants need to grow and thrive. In this sense, all formulas are "the same." Every infant formula sold in the US is required by the Food and Drug Administration (FDA) to meet the nutrient levels set forth in the Infant Formula Act of 1980. As a result, all infant formulas provide largely the same nutrition, offering protein, fat, carbohydrates, vitamins, and minerals at a similar level.

Given this, how is a parent supposed to choose between the twenty-five or more formula options on the market? It can feel overwhelming! I suggest using a three-tiered framework:

First, learn about the ingredients used in formula and decide which ingredients you want to prioritize. Know that what makes one formula different from another is the ingredients list—those foods used to source many of the included nutrients—not the quantity of vitamins and minerals listed on the label.

Second, consider what sort of unique needs your baby has that may inform the type of formula that will work best for them. More on this later!

Third, consider what is important to you—the parent—when it comes to your baby's formula. There are no right or wrong answers here. You should consider price, availability, quality indicators, preferred ingredients, and more.

Let's go through this process together.

Ingredients

As ingredients offer the primary differences between formulas, parents need to know what to look for when it comes to a formula's ingredient list. Formula ingredients fall into two categories: macronutrients (proteins, carbs, fats) and micronutrients (vitamins and minerals). You need to know about both!

Macronutrients

Proteins

There are a variety of protein sources that can be used in infant formula per FDA regulations. These include cow milk protein, goat milk protein, soy protein, whey protein concentrate, protein hydrolysates (such as casein hydrolysate or partially or extensively hydrolyzed whey protein), and amino acids. Many formulas will contain more than one protein type! The great majority of infants can tolerate a "routine" or "standard" formula, meaning one that contains *intact* milk proteins from either cow's milk or goat's milk. That's right! Because most infants do well on a cow's milk–based formula, infants may not require a partially hydrolyzed, or "gentle," formula to start. Although both routine and gentle formulas are considered safe, there isn't compelling data to suggest that gentle formulas should be used routinely.

While often used as a base for infant formula, cow's milk and goat's milk alone aren't identical to human milk when it comes to protein structure. For example, mature breast milk contains roughly 60 percent whey protein and roughly 40 percent casein protein, referred to as a 60:40 whey-to-casein ratio. Breast milk also includes a type of beta-casein protein similar to the A2 beta-casein that's found in abundance in other mammal milks. Cow's milk, on the other hand, contains roughly 20 percent whey protein and roughly 80 percent casein protein (an 80:20 ratio), and most commonly includes both A1 and A2 beta-casein protein types. As a result of these differences, some manufacturers develop infant formulas with cow's milk as a base and then include additional whey protein, which makes the whey-to-casein ratio more similar to that found in mature breast milk, or milk produced beginning fourteen days or so after birth. Formulas with added whey protein (often listed as "whey protein concentrate" in the ingredients list) and those that use milk with solely or predominantly A2 proteins are more reflective of the protein structure of human milk.

Tl;dr on protein: Healthy, full-term infants usually start with a formula that uses cow's milk as the base. Formulas that include extra whey protein, A2 proteins, or partially hydrolyzed (a.k.a. broken-down) proteins, if needed, can support digestion.

Carbohydrates

Babies need a lot of carbs to sustain their rapid growth—carbohydrates make up roughly 40 percent of the calories that come from breast milk or infant formula! Carbohydrates in infant formula typically come from one or more sources, including lactose (a sugar found naturally in mammal milks), maltodextrin, sucrose, corn syrup or corn syrup solids, or tapioca starch. Any of these ingredients can provide the carbs infants need to grow appropriately. It's also worth noting that the corn syrup used in some infant formulas is *not* high-fructose corn syrup.

For parents looking for a formula that's "close to breast milk," lactose is the ideal carbohydrate source. Why? Because the principal energy-contributing carbohydrate source in breast milk is lactose! This is true *regardless* of whether the lactating parent consumes dairy. Lactose is inherent at high levels in human milk among all lactating individuals, even those who have cut milk products from their diet. Babies begin producing lactase, an enzyme that digests lactose, while in utero (in the second and third trimester). This means that babies are biologically designed to digest lactose. As a result, nearly all full-term infants can consume lactose in breast milk and/or formula. The rare exception are infants born with congenital lactase deficiency, galactosemia, or other medical conditions impacting digestion of lactose.

While lactose is ideal as a carbohydrate in baby formula, all carb sources used in FDA-regulated infant formulas have been clinically studied and proven safe for use. Some infants who have a cow's milk protein allergy will require a formula that is lactose-free, and others may simply do better on a reduced-lactose or lactose-free formula. I used a reduced-lactose formula for my first baby and wouldn't hesitate to do so again if my baby tolerated it better! Alternative carbohydrate sources shouldn't give parents pause.

Tl;dr on carbs: Lactose-based formulas are ideal and appropriate for the great majority of healthy, term infants, though alternatives are also safe.

Fats

All regulated infant formulas in the US, Canada, and Europe contain seed oils. Wild, right? This fact often creates concern among parents who try to avoid seed oils or vegetable oils in their own diets. But the truth is, breast milk has a unique mix of fatty acids that differs from the fats found in cow's milk or goat's milk, and therefore it is not possible to use only cow's or goat's milk fat as the source of fat in infant formula. It's important to remember that infants are not tiny adults, and their nutrient needs differ dramatically from ours due to their rapid rate of growth. Because the fatty acid profile of cow's milk and goat's milk does not mirror that of human milk, plant-based oils are added (occasionally along with milk fat) to provide the essential fatty acids infants need to grow.

Typically, infant formulas include sunflower or safflower oil (a source of oleic and linoleic fatty acids), coconut oil (a source of lauric acid), and one or more of soybean oil, palm or palm olein oil, or low–erucic acid rapeseed oil, also known as canola oil (all of which provide oleic, linoleic, and palmitic acid, among others). Currently, olive oil, avocado oil, grapeseed oil, or other fat sources such as tallow and cocoa butter are not authorized for use as sources of fat in infant formula in the US. These fat sources have not been through the appropriate regulatory process to ensure that they've been studied for safety, efficacy, or shelf stability for use in infant formula at this point.

Plant-based oils in formula provide essential fatty acids such as omega-3s and omega-6s that are inherent in breast milk. They're also a source of necessary calories. Without essential fatty acids, an infant could suffer from malnutrition in the form of essential fatty acid deficiency! Truly, plant-based oils are necessary in infant formula. For parents who want to minimize common concerns around vegetable oil sourcing and processing (whether that's pesticide use on crops, chemical solvents used for extraction, or bleaching agents used to reduce color—all of which are commercially safe for use), choosing a formula with organic oils is recommended.

Tl;dr on oils: All infant formulas have plant-based oils because they need them. You want these oils in your baby's formula, as they help to mirror the fatty acid composition in breast milk and they promote healthy growth.

Micronutrients

Vitamins and Minerals

All infant formulas sold in the US must contain certain micronutrients within certain ranges based on a one-hundred-calorie serving size. As a result, the amount of each micronutrient is similar across formula products. Two micronutrients to pay attention to that sometimes differ from product to product:

- *Vitamin D:* The amount of vitamin D in a serving of your baby's formula will tell you whether you need to offer an additional daily vitamin D supplement. The AAP recommends 400 IU daily throughout the first year! If your baby's formula intake doesn't provide 400 IU of vitamin D daily, based on the amount per serving in their formula and how much formula they consume per day, you should supplement.

- *Iron:* The overall average concentration of iron in US infant formulas is 1.8 mg of iron per 100-calorie serving, although a few infant formulas contain less at 1.0 mg or 1.2 mg per serving. If your baby is at higher-than-average risk of iron deficiency or iron deficiency anemia or is partially or fully breastfed, your pediatrician may recommend a formula with iron content on the higher end or an oral iron supplement.

TL;dr on micronutrients: They're pretty much the same across products.

Extras

Because all infant formulas contain the same required nutrients in largely the same amounts, brands often include non-FDA-required ingredients to differentiate themselves in a crowded market. These include DHA and ARA (types of fatty acids), lactoferrin (a type of protein), a source of milk fat globule membrane (MFGM), human milk oligosaccharides (HMOs, a type of prebiotic), galactooligosaccharides or fructooligosaccharides (GOS or FOS, types of prebiotics), probiotics ("good bacteria"), and alpha-lactalbumin whey (a type of protein), among others. These components exist in breast milk, but most have limited or mixed clinical significance when added to infant formula. I call these "nice-to-have extras," because while they are safe for infants, the FDA has not determined they are crucial for infant health or development.

Tl;dr on extras: Don't break your budget for ingredients that aren't required unless you really want them.

Just Tell Me Which Formula to Pick, Please!

I wish I could! Choosing a formula, however, requires sorting through a variety of considerations that are unique to your family. Here's where the second and third parts of our "picking a formula framework" come into play:

> *Does this formula meet my baby's needs?*

and

> *Does this formula align with my priorities and values as a parent?*

So many parents focus only on the former criterion and then wonder why they feel so bad about using formula. By weighing the latter criterion just as heavily, parents can choose a formula that *everyone* in the family feels good using.

Factors to consider on baby's end include the baby's gestational age at birth (premature infants often require a dedicated preemie formula with extra calories!), their digestive symptoms (would a thickened formula for reflux be beneficial?), and their medical conditions (e.g., to accommodate an allergy or a condition that affects nutrient absorption).

Factors to consider on the parents' end include availability, cost, quality indicators (e.g., is grass-fed milk important to you?), religious or cultural factors that may influence ingredient preferences or restrictions, and brand values.

Identifying these criteria and comparing them across products can help narrow down the field to those formulas that will fit your needs. See the chart below, circle what resonates for your family, and then bring it to your pediatrician—they can help identify formulas that meet your criteria! And remember, no formula choice is permanent. You can always try something different if the first one isn't a fit.

I recommend giving your baby at least seven to ten days on a formula before switching (provided there's no evidence of allergy or intolerance), as sometimes it takes their brand-new digestive systems some time to adjust. Every baby is different, so if you're not sure if a formula is a fit for your child, be sure to reach out to your child's health care professional for guidance.

Parent Preferences for Formula

Cost	Availability	Certifications	Ingredients
WIC-covered	Online—subscription	USDA organic	Includes DHA/ARA
~$0.50 / ounce	Online—non-subscription	EU organic	Includes prebiotics (HMOs, GOS, FOS)
~$1.00 / ounce	Online—Amazon	Non-GMO	Avoids soy
~$1.50 / ounce	Retail—grocery	Kosher	Avoids palm and/or palm olein oil
~$2.00 / ounce	Retail—club store	Halal	Avoids corn syrup
No cost concern	Retail—pharmacy	Vegetarian	Avoids maltodextrin
	Delivery—Instacart	Clean Label Project	Contains added whey protein
			Contains A2 proteins

6

Getting Over the Guilt

Making the decision to use formula—or needing to use it due to circumstances beyond your control—can be emotionally fraught. So many moms express *feeling bad* about it. There is so much to unpack with those two words that it would take another book—and a qualified mental health expert—to excavate it. I can't tell you why you feel bad or what to do about it, but I can tell you why *I* felt bad and what helped me move past it. Hopefully it will resonate with you.

When I introduced formula and then switched to exclusively formula feeding, I felt bad about it for a number of reasons. First, I felt bad for disappointing people. I'm a people pleaser at heart, and I thrive on following rules, meeting people's expectations, and being rewarded for it with their praise.

Feeling like I let everyone down (my obstetrician, my child's pediatrician, my husband, my baby!) was acutely difficult for me, especially after I had previously told them my plans and then didn't follow through on them.

Second, I felt bad for "not giving my baby the best." I knew, after doing the research and attending the classes, that breast milk offered ideal nutrition for my baby. And what parent *doesn't* want what's ideal for their newborn? I felt bad that I couldn't provide that for her, and I worried she'd be worse off for life because of it. You've likely seen the scare tactics and statistics that make formula feeding seem like a life sentence for bad health.

Third, I felt bad because I *didn't* feel bad. That's some messed-up stuff, I know, but I felt bad because giving up breastfeeding made me feel relieved. I thought something was fundamentally wrong with me, because while I felt like a disappointment and a failure (see points one and two), I didn't feel *sad* about the end of our breastfeeding journey. I was grateful, and I felt bad about it.

Lastly, I felt bad because I had been conditioned to believe I *was* bad for feeding my child formula. I had been exposed to endless commentary on social media that called formula feeding selfish, that minimized and invalidated my struggles with breast milk supply, that promoted self-sacrifice at any cost to keep nursing, and that labeled formula as "poison." No wonder I felt bad! I now know that this is often the point. Some pro-breastfeeding groups, lactivists, and even well-meaning public health communications lean into these ideas because a mom refusing formula is a win in their book—no matter if it took the purposeful manipulation of her feelings during a vulnerable time to get there.

So with all of this at play, I felt bad. Like, *bad* bad. "Maybe I wasn't cut out to be a mother" kind of bad. And while I don't think the struggles I had with breastfeeding and the guilt and shame I felt about formula feeding caused my postpartum depression with my first child, they certainly did nothing to help.

When I look back, I can't identify a single action that made the biggest difference in getting over the guilt, but I can identify several that pushed me in a better direction. Some of these may be helpful tools for you:

- *Therapy:* I had been in and out of therapy for years (again, I'm a recovering people pleaser and perfectionist—my issues started long before I had kids!), but I made the decision to go back to therapy on a weekly basis a few months after my daughter was born. Because she was on formula, I was able to have someone else stay with her while I attended! We talked through so many of my feelings about our feeding journey, and I did EMDR therapy for some particularly sticky, negative moments I had while pumping. To be honest, I *still* uncover the occasional lingering negative feeling about breastfeeding, formula, and my postpartum journey in therapy these days. If you have access to it, counseling with a professional can be a great place to start working through your feelings.

- *Medication:* Like counseling, I had been on an anti-depressant medication at certain times before I had kids. When I couldn't get out of the constant, intrusive, mental berating of myself for my own uselessness postpartum (it's not always fun in my brain, y'all), I decided—along with my primary care doctor and my husband's encouragement—to get back on medication and then later to increase my dose. It was 100 percent the right choice for me in that season, and it continued to be the right choice for me during my pregnancy with my son and beyond. I know it can be scary thinking about pharmaceutical help for intrusive thoughts or challenging mental health, but it's worth a discussion with your doctor if you can't get out of negative thought cycles no matter what you do.

- *Research Deep Dive:* I mentioned in the intro to this book that I'm a researcher (at one point professionally and now casually). Something that was dramatically helpful in easing my negative feelings about not breastfeeding was digging into the high-quality research about short- and long-term outcomes of breastfed and formula-fed infants. While there isn't as much data as we'd all like (because it's unethical to run a double-blind randomized control trial where you force half the group to feed one way and half the group to feed the other), there are still some good studies that show the long-term differences between formula-fed and breastfed infants are much smaller

than they're typically portrayed online. My favorite
resource here is the book *Cribsheet* by Emily Oster,
an economist at Brown University who is brilliant at
analyzing data and distilling it for the nonscientists
among us. She has an entire chapter in *Cribsheet* that
looks at the research on breastfeeding versus formula
feeding, and it helped me put into better perspective
what I thought I was "depriving my daughter of" by
not nursing.

• *Understanding Risk:* The handout my ob-gyn's office
gave me about feeding a baby had a lot of claims
about formula feeding. It read something like,
"Formula-fed infants are twice as likely to be diagnosed with [ear infections, type 1 diabetes, insert
whatever other scary condition you've heard about
here] compared to breastfed infants." Yikes, right?
This sort of statistic understandably creates concern—
no parent wants to double their baby's risk for a
medical condition, particularly one that's painful (or
lifelong). What I didn't know then, but know now, is
that this type of risk assessment is called *relative risk*.
It shares the probability of an event occurring for one
group compared to another group—provided the
second group is not engaging in the same behavior as
the first. Breastfeeding promotional materials often
highlight relative risk. What's missing, in order for
parents to truly make informed feeding decisions, is a
discussion of *absolute risk*, or the overall probability of

something occurring in a defined group or individual. To make a true risk assessment, we have to understand not just relative risk but also absolute risk. For example, what if formula feeding doubles your baby's risk, but the absolute risk has gone from 0.02 percent to 0.04 percent? Yes, the risk is doubled, but not meaningfully; in this example, there's a 99.96 percent chance of no event occurring regardless of how you feed. Understanding this nuance helped me view those scary statistics much more objectively!

- *Milestone Tracking:* I use *milestone* loosely here because I don't mean the typical developmental milestones like waving or crawling. What helped me get over the guilt of using formula was watching my kids thrive on it. Formula helped my first baby go from struggling to gain weight to consistently gaining. She was a more content baby. We started to bond so much more. She started to love her bottle. Watching all of this unfold—and really paying attention to it and appreciating it—helped me feel better about formula. After all, how could I feel bad about something that was making our lives (and our health) so much better?

- *Reality Checking:* Sometimes the answer is tough love, and for me, this looked like my mom stating, "I formula fed you, and you turned out exceptionally well." While "exceptionally" may be a bit extreme, I can acknowledge that there's no part of me that wishes I had been breastfed or wonders if I may have been smarter or healthier if I had been.

The reality is that the majority of babies in the US are fed formula at some point, and in previous decades, the number was even more significant than it is today. Statistically, this means there are Olympians, Nobel laureates, astronauts, CEOs, neurosurgeons, presidents and prime ministers, and any other manner of people with impressive résumé credentials who were formula fed. We can't know for sure, though, because no one asks these people how they were fed as infants. *Because it doesn't matter as adults.* Because there are other factors that are more relevant and more interesting that matter more. (And of course, your baby doesn't have to grow up to be exceptional according to worldly standards to make formula feeding a valid choice. The knowledge that formula-fed babies *can* grow up to be exceptional was enough to help the guilt for me.)

- *Time:* The last piece of the puzzle for me was time. While I don't believe that time heals all wounds, the older your children get, the less you're likely to worry about your feeding journey in infancy. During your baby's first year of life, this one decision feels like *the most important* decision. With a bit of time and perspective, it's easier to see clearly that it's just one in a long line of decisions. You will wake up one day— three, five, ten years from now—to realize you can't remember the last time you gave a second thought as to how you fed your baby. Time shifts importance to what needs to be addressed *now*, and with it, guilt about how you addressed needs *then* falls away.

As I said before, I can't tell you how to get over any bad feelings you may have about using formula. For you, talking to a friend, working out your thoughts on a run, or removing social media from your phone might be the answer. No matter what, I encourage you to do the work of trying *something*. You deserve to enjoy your baby's first year without being bogged down in negative feelings about yourself or your choices. I want that for you, and I want you to want this—and know you deserve it—for yourself.

Quick Tip:
How to Set Up a Feeding Station

Babies, like adults, aren't patient when they are hungry! The best way to avoid a hangry baby is to set up a feeding station: a designated place to keep the items you need for feeding so bottles can be assembled quickly and safely. If the parent's bedroom or baby's bedroom is on a separate floor from the kitchen, I recommend setting up a feeding station on both levels. No one wants to stumble down the stairs at three o'clock in the morning to make a bottle! Here's what to include (ideally in a space that is distinct from cooking prep areas to reduce the risk of contamination):

- A few clean, dry bottles and nipples. Keep them unassembled so you don't have to break them apart before you prep the bottle!

- Formula—either the full container or preportioned powder in a clean formula dispenser according to feeding volume.

- Whatever water you use to mix with powdered or concentrate formula in a sealed container. Check with your pediatrician to confirm whether they recommend boiled and cooled water, room temperature tap water, or gallons of purified or distilled water!

- Burp cloths. I suggest at least two, but the more the better.

- A pacifier to keep your baby occupied in case you need to make additional ounces of formula mid-feeding.

- A bin to hold used bottles when the feeding is

done (if you're not near your sink). A Tupperware
container or other plastic receptacle without the
lid works great!

· A change of clothes for baby—diaper and wipes,
plus a onesie or sleeper.

· Vitamin D drops if your baby is drinking less than
thirty-two ounces of formula per day, based on
AAP recommendations of 400 IU per day through
the first year.

· (Optional) A small, dorm-size mini-fridge. This can
be a great addition to a bedroom feeding station
and can be used to keep prepared bottles cold
until ready for use, or to keep expressed milk cold
after pumping.

· (Optional) A bottle warmer if you choose to use one.

Having these materials organized makes it quick
and easy to prep a bottle and serve within minutes.
I suggest restocking the feeding station every night
before you go to bed so it's ready to go when you
need it (either overnight or in the morning). While it
sounds like a simple, commonsense strategy to put all
your feeding supplies in one place, it can be a game
changer for reducing stress during feeding times.

Mom Note
Leave Your House!

When my first child was a newborn, even thinking about leaving the house left me in a cold sweat (okay, it might've been the hormones, too; postpartum sweating is no joke)! It just seemed too difficult—too many unknowns to think through and make plans for, too much stuff to bring in the diaper bag, too little control over traffic or wait times at the coffee shop, too many strangers who might want to touch my baby with their germy hands. Getting out of the house can feel like a lot when you're a new parent. Plus, there are plenty of tasks to keep you busy *without* leaving home during the postpartum season: dishes, laundry, nap times, meal prep, cleaning the kitchen . . . it can feel easier to just hunker down.

There's nothing wrong with this, especially in the early days with a new baby! But I encourage you, especially if you're feeling isolated or blue, not to stay stuck for too long. In my opinion, the best way to feel like a real human, outside of your role as a parent to a new baby, is to leave your house. Why? Because that's where all the other humans are human-ing.

I'm not suggesting you go wild and bring your baby to the mall. (If you want to, more power to you! We brought our second child to a mariachi restaurant when he was a week old.) You can start small. Don't go far, and don't go for long. Here are a few suggestions for getting out of the house that may feel manageable:

- Sit on the back porch (or in your driveway, or in your parked car) in a sunbeam for a few minutes.

- Drive through McDonald's and get an ice cream cone (and pray on the way that the machine isn't broken).

- Put your baby in their crib (alone—no blankets or stuffed animals!) and go check the mail.

- Take the stroller for a walk in a local park.

- Drop off your dry cleaning.

- If you have a partner or friend that works outside the home, bring them lunch. You don't have to stay!

- Check out a local "baby & me" group in your community.

Like everything, the more you get out with (or without) your new baby, the more confident you'll become. Staying connected to the world and the people around you, even in these small ways, can be a balm to the loneliness that many of us feel postpartum. If it feels like the world has continued to rotate beyond you and without you, try leaving your house. Put yourself back into the comings and goings of your community. I can't promise it will always be easy or fun (your baby is bound to have a meltdown or diaper blowout at some point), but I can promise it helps.

7

How to Make a Bottle (and How to Make Your Life Easier)

In 2024, the Centers for Disease Control and Prevention shared information about a longitudinal study that found that out of four thousand women surveyed, only *12 percent had been instructed by a health care provider on how to make a bottle of formula* by the time their baby was two months old. This is abysmal, especially as three-quarters of US parents aren't exclusively breastfeeding by the time their baby turns six months old. A baby's health depends on safe and accurate bottle preparation. Here's how to do it correctly!

The first step to making a bottle is always the same: *Wash your hands*. Always wash your hands before touching bottle parts, the bottle nipple, the lid on your formula container, the scoop, and any other feeding equipment. Washing your hands is important to reduce the likelihood of introducing bacteria to your baby's bottle. This is especially important, as infants have brand-new, immature immune systems and are more susceptible to infections than older children and adults. To wash effectively:

1. Use warm water and regular soap (no need for antibacterial soap).

2. Scrub for at least twenty seconds.

3. Rinse your hands.

4. Dry them thoroughly—we don't want to risk introducing moisture to your container of powdered formula.

Once you have clean hands, the steps for making a bottle will differ depending on the format of the formula you're using. While general guidelines will be shared below, always defer to the mixing instructions on your container of formula, as they account for any differences across products (like scoop size or suggested water temperature).

Liquid Ready-to-Feed Formula

This one is easy-peasy! If you're using a two-ounce ready-to-feed bottle, sometimes called a *nurser*, simply screw on the disposable collar and nipple that the brand sells alongside these newborn formula bottles. You don't have to transfer the formula to a different bottle if you don't want to. If you'd prefer to use your own bottle (if, for example, you only want to use half the nurser and save the other half in the fridge for later), pour from the two-ounce bottle into your own *without adding any additional water*. Liquid ready-to-feed formula does not need to be diluted or reconstituted with additional water!

Liquid ready-to-feed formulas also come in larger sizes that typically contain eight or thirty-two ounces. These can be poured from and then capped before storing in the fridge and will remain good for up to forty-eight hours after opening or according to the label's storage instructions. Never transfer liquid ready-to-feed formula into any other container besides your baby's bottles.

Water Break!

Before getting into the specifics of how to make a bottle using liquid concentrate or powdered infant formula, we need to talk about water—specifically, the type of water that can and cannot be used and the recommended temperature of the water. First, know that different public health agencies offer different guidance on this topic depending on the population they serve. The American Academy of Pediatrics, which serves the US, offers different advice from the World Health Organization, which operates globally. This is because the US has the Environmental Protection Agency (EPA), which sets standards and regulations for clean water. The Centers for Disease Control and Prevention and the Food and Drug Administration offer different guidance as well. Your best bet for identifying the appropriate water type and temperature for your baby is to discuss with your pediatrician, as they know your baby's needs best. Always use water from a safe source!

Types of water that are typically recommended include:

- Tap water (if safe to drink in your area—check with your local health department if you're unsure)

- Distilled water

- Purified water

Types of water that are typically not recommended for daily formula consumption include:

- Tap water (if unsafe to drink or if there is uncertainty about safety)

- Well water (if the safety of water from a private well is compromised)

Some pediatricians suggest boiling the water (tap, distilled, or purified) for one minute and letting it cool for five minutes before mixing with formula, as this kills off any potential bacteria or microbes that could cause illness. The FDA recommends this for infants who were born prematurely, infants who are immunocompromised, and newborns under the age of two months. Always check the temperature of the formula before serving to ensure it's not too hot; placing a few drops on the inside of the wrist is an ideal method! Formula should be served no cooler than refrigerator temperature (approximately 37 degrees Fahrenheit) and no hotter than body temperature (98–100 degrees Fahrenheit).

Liquid Concentrate Formula

Unlike liquid ready-to-feed formula, liquid concentrate formula *does* need to be diluted with water. Failure to dilute concentrated formula can endanger your baby's health! As a rule of thumb, formula concentrate typically comes in cans while ready-to-feed formula comes in plastic bottles or cartons. Double-checking the type of liquid formula you have on hand by reading the label before using is always a good idea.

After washing your hands, shake the can vigorously to mix the contents. If the can has a pull tab, use that to remove the top. If there is no pull tab, use a clean can opener. A punch-type can opener is recommended. Next, pour equal amounts of water and formula into your baby's bottle. Liquid concentrate formula uses a one-to-one ratio: one part formula for every one part water (for example, two ounces of water and two ounces of liquid concentrate formula if making a four-ounce bottle).

Once added, shake to mix as directed on the can. Liquid concentrate formula includes stabilizers to prevent ingredients from separating, and they also make it less likely to foam when mixed.

Generally speaking, formula left in the can should be covered, stored in the refrigerator, and used within forty-eight hours of opening. Unopened cans should be stored in a cool, dry place away from extreme temperatures, like a pantry or upper cabinet. Be sure to read label guidance, though, in case specific preparation or storage instructions vary from one brand of liquid concentrate to another.

Powdered Formula

Water is needed to reconstitute powdered formula into a liquid product. Here are the steps you need to know:

1. Add water to your bottle before the powder. This helps ensure an accurate ratio of powder to water, which will allow the mixture to meet the nutrition facts on the back panel of the container! You should add as much water as the volume of formula you intend to make (i.e., if you want to make four ounces of formula, add four ounces of water to the bottle).

2. Add the correct number of level scoops of powder. While many powdered formulas use a one-to-two ratio—one scoop for every two ounces of water— some use a one-to-one ratio. Consult the instructions on your formula container to confirm! Take the scoop included with the formula and fill it with

powder. You can give the scoop one or two gentle taps to eliminate any large pockets of air. Unless otherwise advised on the formula's label, repeated tapping is not recommended, as this can cause the formula to pack, and most powdered formulas require unpacked scoops. Use a clean, flat utensil (like a knife) or the side of the can or container to level the scoop, removing any extra powder from the top. Add the powder to the water.

3. Replace the scoop in the formula container and close the lid! Store the formula container as recommended on the container's label. It is recommended to store the container in a cool, dry place (but not in the refrigerator).

4. Mix the formula (check out the Quick Tip next for my favorite strategy here). Serve immediately or store in the fridge and use within twenty-four hours if serving later.

Note that unopened powdered formula should be stored in a cool, dry environment. Opened powdered formula must be used within a month of opening.

Formula Food Safety Rules

Formula is food, and just like we have rules about how long other animal-based food products can sit out at room temperature or chill in the fridge, there are also rules for formula. While the formula container's instructions for storage are the ultimate recommendation for how to keep your formula safe, as a general rule of thumb, remember 24:2:1.

24 hours: Powdered formula that has been prepared but not served is good in the refrigerator for up to twenty-four hours. Some parents prefer to make a day's worth of formula in one batch for the sake of convenience, while others prep a few bottles for the fridge. Several brands offer formula-mixing pitchers, which allow for formula batching! A pitcher with prepared formula can be stored in the fridge and used to pour from as needed when it's time for a feeding, provided it's used or discarded within twenty-four hours of preparation.

2 hours: Powdered formula that has been prepared but not served is good at room temperature for up to two hours.

1 hour: Prepared formula, no matter the format, that has been offered to your baby should be discarded one hour after the start of the feeding.

The purpose of these food safety rules is to reduce the likelihood that bacteria introduced to the formula (during the prep process or from your baby's mouth) can multiply to a level that causes contamination. Given that babies are more susceptible to illness than most, following these rules provides the best chance for reducing the likelihood of sickness.

Making Bottles at Night

Three in the morning is not the time to figure out how to make a bottle! Use the following tricks to make bottle prep and feeding easier overnight:

- Some parents prefer to use liquid ready-to-feed formula at night, even when using powder or liquid concentrate formula during the day. Removing the need to measure and mix at night can save time and frustration!

- If using powdered or concentrate formula, pour the correct volume of water into bottles (but do not add the powdered or liquid concentrate formula at this point), cap the bottles, and keep them in your room or baby's room. These can be kept at room temperature until you are ready to add the powder or liquid concentrate for the middle-of-the-night feedings! I recommend having one or two extra bottles filled with water compared to what you think you will need. You can always use them the next day if you don't need them at night.

- Preportion powdered formula into clean, single-serving containers to keep next to the bottles filled with the appropriate volume of water.

- Acclimate your baby to room temperature bottles during the day to save the step of warming them up overnight.

- Prep mixed bottles ahead of time and keep them in a mini-fridge in your room or baby's room. A dorm-size fridge can be a game changer for bottles overnight!

- If your baby demands a warm bottle (instead of room temperature or cold from the fridge), it's often faster and easier to place the bottle in a mug of hot water from the sink than it is to use a conventional bottle warmer. Keep a mug by your sink for this purpose.

- If your baby demands a warm bottle quickly and you're using powdered or liquid concentrate formula, consider purchasing an electric hot water dispenser or an electric kettle. Another option is to keep warm water in a clean thermos until it's ready to be used. Remember to always test the temperature of the formula before serving.

Quick Tip:
Stirred, Not Shaken
(or, How to Reduce Bubbles)

You've assembled your baby's bottle! Now it's time to mix it. The most common way to dissolve powdered formula in water is to shake the bottle, and that's what most formula labels' preparation instructions recommend. But that may not be the *smartest* way. Two reasons for this:

1. Most parents will intuitively put their thumb over the bottle's nipple to pinch it closed so the formula doesn't spray everywhere and make a mess while shaking. While effective at preventing a mess, if parents skipped the step of cleaning their hands first, this can allow bacteria on the thumb to migrate to the nipple and/or into the milk. We want to avoid this!

2. While shaking a bottle works well to dissolve powdered formula, the significant agitation that comes from shaking can cause bubbles and/or a layer of foam to form on top of the milk. As much as possible, we want to reduce the likelihood that our baby will swallow extra air, as this can potentially lead to gas and discomfort. Think about drinking a carbonated beverage yourself—bubbles in your drink cause gas and burping! Fewer bubbles in the bottle can mean less gas in the belly.

Instead of shaking to mix, I suggest gently swirling the mixture or stirring it with a clean utensil. Using warm water can also increase solubility, requiring less agitation to get the mixture to dissolve.

If you want or need to shake the bottle to mix, place a clean cap over the nipple (instead of your finger!) and, if possible, allow for the bottle to sit for several minutes before feeding so that some of the foam can break up.

Mom Note
Find Little Luxuries

When a new baby enters the home, parents' wants and needs tend to take a back seat. For good reason! Your new baby has no capacity to care for itself. You, however, do—and it's important not to inadvertently neglect yourself during those upside-down newborn weeks. I personally found it difficult to know what "self-care" looked like in that season. I couldn't exercise, I couldn't travel, I couldn't enjoy a glass of wine (on account of C-section-related painkillers and, after, my medication for postpartum depression), and I didn't have the ability to schedule a last-minute meetup with a friend. I barely had the energy to keep my eyes open long enough to read, and social media scrolling made me feel worse instead of better. I was stuck in a loop of giving and giving and giving of myself without anything to refill my own cup, and it left me wrung out and half-dead. I wasn't the parent I wanted to be when feeling like that.

Enter: the little luxury. What works in the postpartum season is finding and appreciating self-care on a *micro level*.

These are tiny indulgences that exist just for you and for your enjoyment of them. Here are some ideas I used and loved:

- A hot towel to drape over the neck and shoulders to ease the ache of all those hours hunched over feeding the baby

- A nice piece of dark chocolate

- A cheap arrangement of flowers from the grocery store (or cut from the yard)

- A three-minute dance break to a favorite song

- Watching or listening to a comedy clip on YouTube—laughter is such a good mood booster!

- A special drink (alcoholic or not)

- Aromatherapy oils, a nice candle, or a room spray in a favorite scent

- Sitting in the car with a sleeping baby in the back while the sun warms the front seat

- Salt scrub for a bath or shower

- A podcast to listen to while washing bottles or doing laundry

- A standing phone call with a good friend each week or month

- A fuzzy blanket to sit under when baby naps

- Anything else that brings you joy and is quick and easy

You may have noticed a theme in these suggestions: Most of them provide a sensory experience. They offer a flavor, scent, sound, or feeling, and I find this to be grounding, especially during times of stress. The newborn season can be overstimulating—so much crying, so much touching, so many smells! Reclaiming the senses for your own momentary pleasure is an easy way to stay connected to who you are outside of your role as a parent.

It may seem like small potatoes (i.e., "*Your expert advice is to suggest I sit under a blanket?*"), but finding, acknowledging, and appreciating moments of little luxury can be wildly meaningful during a season that offers little self-care otherwise. Try it before you knock it!

8

Position Matters
(When It Comes to Feeding)

While breastfeeding comes with many position suggestions (rugby or football hold, side-lying, cross-cradle, and
more), most parents assume there is only one position for
bottle feeding. Typically, this looks like a reclined baby
with their neck in the crook of a caregiver's elbow and the
bottle at a forty-five-degree angle to their mouth. Something like this:

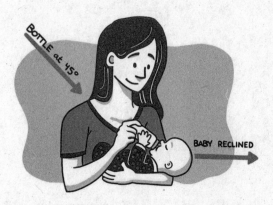

This position above is what parents tend to see out and about, at Mommy and Me classes, and in popular media. But this position is not always the ideal bottle feeding position, especially for new babies. Instead, we want to position the baby more like this:

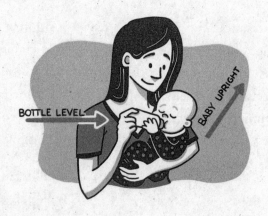

In this position, the baby is relatively upright, and the bottle is horizontal—or level—with the baby's mouth. A similar position is called *side-lying*, which looks like this position below. Notice how the bottle is still level with the baby's mouth!

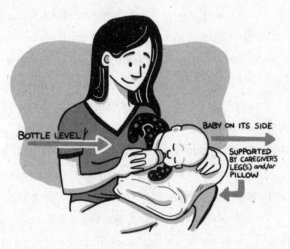

BOTTLE LEVEL

BABY ON ITS SIDE

SUPPORTED BY CAREGIVER'S LEG(S) and/or PILLOW

To understand why position matters, let's start with a thought experiment. Imagine that you are lying flat on your back, on the floor, with an open bottle of water in your hand. Imagine lifting the water bottle to your mouth to drink while lying flat. You may immediately anticipate the problem: Gravity will cause the water to dump on your face, and there will be no way to control the flow. In this thought experiment, you can almost feel the anxiety that would come from trying to catch a breath while the water pours into your mouth and all over your face. You'd likely take big gulps of air whenever you could, not knowing when you might get another break in the flow to breathe. *It is not comfortable for us, as adults, when we cannot control the flow of what we're drinking.*

The same is true for infants!

When a baby is in a reclined position and the bottle is tipped down at an angle, gravity does a lot of the work of pulling the milk down and through the nipple. This is not ideal. We want our babies to do the work of withdrawing the milk from the nipple so that they can control the flow, which also allows them to better coordinate their breathing, sucking, and swallowing. Positioning a baby upright or side-lying while bottle feeding, with the bottle level, more closely mirrors the experience of a baby nursing at the breast. Both require the baby to do the bulk of the work removing milk. This bottle feeding position may also reduce the likelihood of bottle preference for families who are combination feeding or supplementing—a.k.a. switching between bottle and breast—though research is mixed. Studies suggest that these bottle feeding positions, when accompanied by a paced bottle feeding approach, lead to meal durations and feeding rates more similar to breastfeeding.

When a baby has gastrointestinal symptoms like gas or reflux, parents often focus on *what* they are eating: Is there an allergy? An intolerance? Would a different formula help? If breastfeeding, should dietary changes be made? While these questions are valid, it is also important to consider *how* a baby is feeding, positionally. While more data is needed to fully underscore the importance of positioning, making changes to a baby's position to grant them more control of their milk intake by feeding them in an upright position may make a big difference. When it comes to feeding, position matters!

Quick Tip:
Switching Sides

An easy way to promote your baby's gross motor development is by switching the arm used to hold and feed. While nursing parents naturally switch arms while feeding (to empty both breasts), bottle feeding parents tend to always hold the bottle in their dominant hand. This is not ideal!

While feeding, babies like to look up at their caregiver. If a baby is held in the same arm for every feeding, the baby will always turn their neck in the same direction to look up. This can lead to unequal tightness in the neck muscles! By switching your arms (either during a feeding or at alternating feedings), your baby will have the opportunity to stretch both sides of their neck as they look at you. This can help prevent torticollis, which occurs when prolonged muscle contraction in the neck causes the head to tilt unnaturally to one side, as well as positional plagiocephaly, or a flat spot on the head.

Too little brainpower to remember to switch? I get it—newborn sleep deprivation can make you feel like you're in a fog. In this case, ask your partner, childcare provider, or anyone who regularly feeds your baby to always use one arm while you always use the other. Problem solved!

Mom Note
Night Splitting

One of the best benefits of bottle feeding, in my opinion, is that one person isn't solely responsible for feeding the baby or producing the milk. Using formula (or feeding expressed breast milk in a bottle) allows partners, loved ones, friends, and/or babysitters to take part in your baby's feeding journey. This is most helpful, in my opinion, during the night shift. Research is clear that sleep deprivation has a negative impact on mental health, and inversely, getting adequate sleep each night is protective against postpartum depression. I certainly felt this acutely!

My favorite method for maximizing sleep for parents during the newborn stage is a strategy I call *night splitting*. It's as straightforward as it sounds: If you have a partner, family member, or other nighttime help, split the night into equal shifts, and each take half. For us, it worked best to split the evening into a 10:30 p.m.–3:30 a.m. shift and a 3:30 a.m.–8:30 a.m. shift. I typically took the first shift, as I'm more of a night owl by nature, and knowing I had "time off" later in the night to sleep helped my anxiety and stress if my shift with the baby was tough. My husband preferred to take the early-morning shift, as he's an earlier riser, and he felt more comfortable caring for our baby at night after getting five solid hours of sleep.

In talking with friends and fellow parents about this strategy, some prefer to alternate nights versus shifts—some switch every other night, others do two or three nights in a row and then trade off so the opposite partner can really climb out of a sleep deficit with a few good nights strung together. Whatever works for your family and your support system is fine!

A crucial element of night splitting, for many parents, is having the parent who is *not* "on the clock" sleep in a separate space from the baby and on-shift parent. For us, this meant the off-shift parent slept in the primary bedroom and the on-shift parent slept on an air mattress in our baby's nursery. Because here's the deal: Babies can be very noisy when they sleep, and as a new parent, any gurgling or grunting from the bassinet immediately spiked my adrenaline. There was no hope of me sleeping through it if my baby woke up and I was in the room, and I also didn't want the temptation to micromanage my husband (which I was liable to do if I was awake and covertly watching him feed the baby even while I was "off duty").

Splitting the night into two shifts—and thereby guaranteeing each of us at least five hours of uninterrupted sleep each night—was a crucial piece of the puzzle in sustaining my mental health after my second baby was born. While it may not be ideal to spend many nights sleeping separately from a partner, remember that the newborn season is just that—a season—and the name of the game is "do whatever it takes to survive (and maybe get a bit closer to thriving)." For us, night splitting was the answer.

9

What's Normal, What's Not, and When to Switch Formulas

When I had my first baby, I was convinced that if I just found the right formula, or introduced the right probiotic drops, or removed certain things from my diet when I was pumping, or breastfed longer, or used the right bottle or nipple flow, I would have a happier baby. I quickly discovered, however, that none of those things made much of a difference—and goodness knows, I tried (and spent money on!) them all. I couldn't figure out why my baby was as fussy as she was, and I believed there must be an answer out there if I just tried hard enough to figure it out. But even with all my effort, nothing worked. As a result, I felt like a failure.

What I know now is that babies can have digestive issues at times, and it's not always related to what they're eating or how they're eating. Instead, babies may have digestive issues because they have immature digestive systems. Until their digestive systems mature, they may continue to experience occasional digestive symptoms.

Importantly, this is not necessarily a result of anything you are doing or not doing with your baby or their feeding.

There are many reasons why babies have digestive symptoms (regardless of what they eat or how they feed) and these include:

Immaturity: Babies are born with brand-new digestive systems! Their system has never been asked to digest food before. In the womb, babies are fed via the umbilical cord, which operates via the vascular system. The minute a baby is born and they're asked to take food by mouth is the first time their digestive system kicks into gear. Although the human intestine is usually formed anatomically within the first twenty weeks of gestation, functional maturation of the digestive tract—or how it works—develops over time.

Weak esophageal sphincter: This is a ring of muscle at both ends of the esophagus that helps regulate liquid (and later, food) flow. In mature adults, the lower esophageal sphincter helps prevent what goes down to the stomach from coming back up. With new babies, we understand intuitively that they lack muscle coordination—

they can't lift up their heads and can't control their limbs—and this poor muscle function also extends to this muscle in the esophagus. Because this sphincter is weaker in babies than in older children and adults, we tend to see reflux—what goes down can quickly come back up—because the esophageal sphincter isn't strong enough yet to prevent it.

Insufficient digestive enzymes: We know that lactase—the enzyme which breaks down lactose (the primary carbohydrate in breast milk and in many formulas) begins to populate in an infant's gut during the second and third trimesters of pregnancy. Babies that are premature, or even those born early term who have missed several weeks of the third trimester, may not at first have sufficient lactase enzymes in the gut as required to promote effective digestion of lactose.

Gut microbiome: Bacteria in the gut assist digestion by helping to break down food and absorb nutrients. There is disagreement in the scientific community as to whether the infant gut is sterile at birth, and exposure to microbes during birth can vary based on delivery method (vaginal birth versus cesarean section). Either way, infants under the age of one are demonstrated to have lower diversity of gut microbiota compared to other age groups, and this may impact digestion.

The good news is that babies pick up microbes after birth from a variety of sources: from you if you hold your baby on your chest to do skin to skin, if you place your baby on the ground for tummy time, or if you have pets in the home, for example. Babies pick up microbes from their environment, and these microbes help to populate the gut microbiome. As infants get older and come into contact with more microbes in their environment, their gut health and overall nutrition are influenced.

Air intake during feeding: Some babies have trouble coordinating their sucking, swallowing, and breathing while feeding. As adults, we take for granted that we can coordinate these actions relatively seamlessly, although even we sometimes experience a lack of coordination, as evidenced by the experience of something "going down the wrong pipe." Babies who struggle to coordinate sucking, swallowing, and breathing may take in too much air during the feeding process, potentially leading to gas in the belly, which can make them uncomfortable. This trapped gas can also cause reflux as the gas tries to escape and takes some of the liquid volume with it! As infants get older and become more efficient at coordinating these actions, digestive symptoms tend to decrease.

These are some of the reasons why babies experience digestive symptoms from time to time, but exactly which of these symptoms are normal, and for how long? Let's break it down for gas, reflux, infrequent stooling, and occasional bouts of fussiness.

Gas: Parents commonly report gas as a digestive symptom their babies experience. It tends to get better around twelve weeks and continues to improve throughout the first year.

Reflux: Unfortunately, as gas is improving around the three- to four-month mark, reflux tends to get worse. Developmentally, reflux peaks around three months of age and shows some improvement by six months of age, and most cases tend to resolve over the course of the first year. Your baby may follow a different timeline! Generally, reflux often gets worse around the three- to four-month mark for two reasons: volume and positioning.

First, babies are usually taking in more volume at this point compared to earlier in life, as they are requiring more calories but most have not yet started solids. Additionally, babies often become more mobile at this time. Around three months, some babies are starting to roll, have more control over their limbs, and are becoming more interested in their environment. Although the cause of reflux is the poor closure of the lower esophageal sphincter, more volume in the stomach (plus not being in an upright position after feeding) may trigger increased reflux. If you notice increased reflux at this age but your baby is still meeting milestones and is gaining weight appropriately (roughly maintaining their weight percentile), their reflux is likely developmentally normal. See chapter 17 for more on reflux and strategies for managing it!

Infrequent stooling: We'll talk about poop in detail in chapter 10, but it's important to note, as a digestive concern, that the frequency of stooling from one baby to another can vary substantially. It can be normal for a baby to have several bowel movements a day, and it can also be normal for a baby to have a bowel movement every few days. This can be hard for parents to understand, but there are many factors that influence stool frequency: diet and fluid intake, gut microbiome development, ability of the pelvic floor muscles to bear down, and more. If your baby's stool is passed easily without straining, it is not considered constipation even if they have bowel movements infrequently.

There are, however, some digestive symptoms that are abnormal and require a visit to your child's pediatrician to discuss whether further follow-up is required. These include:

- Blood in your baby's stool. Blood or black specks in the stool should always be assessed by your child's doctor. Blood in a baby's stool can be the result of inflammation and irritation in the gut, which can be an indication of an allergy or sensitivity to an ingredient in your baby's diet. If you're concerned about a possible allergy and are not sure if your baby has blood in their stool, ask your pediatrician to run a hemoccult test to look for occult blood that is invisible to the naked eye.

- Projectile vomiting, which is vomiting with volume and force that makes your baby uncomfortable. Most typical infant reflux comes in small amounts, is dribbly (versus forceful), and does not bother a baby. Projectile vomiting should always be assessed by your child's doctor.

- Widespread, pervasive rashes should always be evaluated. While many babies have rashes, including baby acne, which is common and harmless, widespread rashes like hives (and, in some cases, eczema) should be evaluated, as this can be an indication of an allergy and may require further testing.

- Colic, while relatively common in the first few months of infancy, may be an indication of an allergy, although the data remains controversial. Still, if your baby is uncomfortable and traditional soothing methods (see the Quick Tip next!) have not worked, or colic symptoms are continuing beyond twelve weeks, it's worth having a conversation with your pediatrician about whether something else may be at play.

At the end of the day, what's normal for your baby depends on your unique baby. You, as the parent or caregiver, know your baby best! If your baby's symptoms do not seem to be improving, if your baby is uncomfortable (especially after introducing a new formula), or if you feel in your gut like something is off, talk to your pediatrician. That's what they're there for! It's always better to err on the side of caution, and I promise you won't be any more of a frequent flyer at the office than I was.

Quick Tip:
Tools to Soothe a Screamer

My first baby was *not* a happy, smiling, cooing baby. She was a face-twisted-up, beet-red, full-volume screamer. Looking back, she was probably well within the guidelines for a colic diagnosis, but instead of pursuing that answer, I decided her temperament, and overall unhappiness, was because I was doing absolutely everything wrong. Brains are mean sometimes, and the postpartum brain (a.k.a. hormonal and sleep deprived) can be especially cruel. If you're in the same boat, hear me say this: Some babies are just wailers. It doesn't necessarily mean there's an underlying problem that you haven't identified. It doesn't mean you aren't doing the right things. It doesn't mean this is what your baby is going to be like forever (my daughter, at nearly ten years old, is a total delight). And, most importantly, it almost certainly *will* get better with time.

But "giving it time" is hard when you're a new

parent with a screaming baby and you live a thousand lifetimes in every twenty-four-hour period. I've been there, so here are some tried-and-true tips for soothing your baby, adapted from Dr. Harvey Karp's famous Five S's framework, plus a few of my own:

- Wrap that baby up tight ("swaddle").

- Use white noise to emulate familiar sounds from the womb ("shush").

- Place baby on their stomach or side during awake times ("side-lying").

- Place baby in a swing, or hold them in your arms while you gently sway back and forth ("swing").

- Give baby a pacifier or a clean finger to suck on ("suck").

- Bounce with baby on an exercise ball (which is also good for rebuilding core strength, so that's a bonus).

- Do tummy massage: Move between all four quadrants of the abdomen. Some parents like to massage in an "I Love You" pattern, with an *I* along the left side of the body, a reverse *L* on the right side and across the top, and then a *U* from upper left to upper right, sweeping across the bottom.

- Help your baby alternate their legs ("bicycle legs"), which can prompt stubborn gas to move through the digestive system instead of staying trapped in the belly.

- Try a bath or holding your baby's back against the sink and slowly pouring lukewarm water on their scalp.

- Take them outside! Sometimes a change of scenery makes a difference.

- If your baby tolerates the car seat, go for a drive. The movement and hum of the engine can be soothing.

- Try the "football hold": Place your baby with their stomach on your forearm and support their head and neck with your palm, letting their arms and legs dangle.

- Consult with your pediatrician about whether supplements like gas drops, probiotic drops, or gripe water (purified water infused with calming herbs like chamomile or fennel) may help.

Finally, and perhaps most importantly, finding avenues to remove yourself sometimes is a reasonable plan. Did you know that recordings of babies crying incessantly are used as a form of torture? It can be truly maddening, and sometimes what's needed is a break to clear your head and recenter yourself. If you don't have a partner, family in town, or the budget for a babysitter, consider asking someone in your circle who also has a baby to do a swap every once in a while—she watches your baby for a bit (even for fifteen minutes while you decompress in the car or yard outside of her place!), and then you switch.

Excessive crying, whether due to colic or normal development, tends to peak between two and six weeks and typically gets better by three months. If you find something that works for you and your baby during this time, lean in. A win is a win, especially during the fourth trimester.

Mom Note
Guard Your (Social) Feed

It's 2:15 a.m., your baby is eating, and you're struggling to keep your eyes open. What's the obvious plan for staying awake? Your phone. Of course it's your phone! I wouldn't trust anyone who answers differently. Our phones are a one-stop shop for entertainment and connection—something every new mom needs in spades. And yet, I'm here to tell you that your postpartum experience will be better—and your feeding journey will be better—if you *stay off your phone*. Or, at the very least, if you are intentional about the content you consume.

Trust me for a second. I fully see the irony in writing about limiting social media use postpartum when my career as a formula expert relies on women finding me via social media when they're postpartum. But it is this experience of having a platform and being privy to "how the sausage is made," so to speak, that makes me *more* adamant that new moms should protect themselves. Because it's a jungle out there on the interwebs, and there are snakes and vines and gorgeous Janes of the Jungle waiting to trap you (and take your money) if you don't watch where you're stepping. Don't worry—if you keep reading, I'll leave you with ideas of what to do instead when you're alone with your thoughts and seeking connection.

First, the research is clear that social media use during the postpartum period can have a negative impact on new moms' mental health, particularly as it relates to body image and levels of self-criticism. Of course it does! This is as obvious as saying the sky is blue, because social media is a springboard for comparison. Thoughts like the following tend to flow freely:

- How did that mom bounce back so quickly?

- I wish I could produce enough milk to have a freezer stash.

- Gosh, my life would be easier if my partner had six weeks of leave like hers does.

- It really seems like everyone else is figuring this motherhood thing out. Why can't I?

- Is my baby supposed to be holding his bottle by now? Is something wrong with him?

The possibilities for comparison are endless. I'm pretty sure I thought through nearly all of them when I had my babies, and you know what? *Not a single one of those comparisons was productive.* Seeing someone else "bounce back" didn't shame me into bouncing back any sooner than my body allowed. Watching someone stock their freezer full of breast milk didn't increase my own output. Playing a video on loop of a ten-month-old holding a bottle didn't help my son avoid physical therapy for his gross motor delay. Instead, this content (coupled by my inability to create the same outcomes in my own life) reduced my confidence, increased my guilt, and furthered my feelings of being alone in my struggles.

I found myself visiting social media looking for connection and validation but almost always left feeling worse than when I came. You might know the feeling. It's ugly, but if I'm honest, it wasn't *ugly enough* to keep me from opening the apps a bunch of times each day. You might know this feeling, too.

It wasn't until I stopped relying on willpower and started building intentional guardrails that my social media time went down. With less time on social media came less comparison, and with less comparison came a better appreciation for my own life and our unique feeding journey. I want this for you, too!

Here are three key strategies for maintaining a healthy relationship with social media postpartum (and also generally, I've come to discover):

- Occupy your hands and/or brain with something else.

- Make your phone less attractive.

- Figure out what you're asking social media to give you and commit to finding it elsewhere.

The first strategy is the easiest of the three. This is a simple one-to-one swap. If you find yourself scrolling mindlessly during an activity, substitute something else that is not housed on your phone but keeps you occupied (without requiring a ton of brainpower). Some of my personal favorites:

- Read something light or funny on an e-reader.

- Listen to an audiobook.

- Attempt a sudoku puzzle or do a word search.

- Knit, doodle, or color an adult coloring book.

- Mess with a fidget item, like a Slinky, Silly Putty, or a tactile puzzle.

Identifying your alternate activity of choice is only half the battle, however. Next, you need to make the new activity accessible and enticing (keep it where you tend to scroll!) *while also making your phone less accessible and less enticing.* A few ideas:

- Set up screen time limits on your phone to cap the amount of time you can spend on certain apps, and/or limit which apps can be used during certain time frames. For me, every interesting app on my phone shuts down at 10:30 p.m. and doesn't come back to life until 8:30 a.m. Additionally, my social media apps all lock after sixty minutes of use. I had my husband set the passcode so I can't change these settings. Did I beat myself up for "needing someone else to enforce these limits"? For a while. But I stopped once I realized how much happier I was without my typical late-night scrolling. It's okay to use your support system to help you meet your goals!

- Change your phone to gray scale. Phones are dopamine generators. The colors, the light, the endless scroll, the wondering if anything new or exciting has happened since you last checked—this is all purposeful to keep your attention. A great way to make your phone less exciting is to remove the color. You may need to look online for step-by-step instructions on how to do this, but if you have an iPhone, simply go into the Accessibility menu within Settings, find the Display menu, and turn off Color Filters.

- Remove apps from your home screen. I haven't had the Facebook app on my phone for five years. I can still visit Facebook's website on my phone's browser, but simply adding that extra step—forcing myself to seek out the web page versus allowing my thumb to hit the app from muscle memory—has dramatically reduced my use. Similarly, try moving a nonsocial app into the place on your screen where your social media used to be. The time it takes to find the app can be just enough of a pause to evaluate whether you really want to open it.

- Be ruthless in who you follow. Think about your social media experience like a house. You wouldn't let people into your physical living space if they continually made you feel bad, if they bullied or name-called, if they disrespected your choices, or constantly pointed out everything you're doing wrong (and then offered a paid solution to fix it). The same rules apply here. You get to decide who you welcome into your house (which is, in this case, your brain). You don't owe anyone your time or attention! If a person, hashtag, brand, or movement isn't adding to your life or making it better? Cut 'em loose. Your life will move forward even if you never find out whether that influencer's seventh baby is the girl they were praying for or whether your high school sweetheart's new wife got that job. Cut. Them. Loose.

The hardest part, and the part that takes the most time, is utilizing the third strategy: doing the introspective work to identify what you hope to gain from social media and then committing to finding it elsewhere. Personally, I seek out social media for a few things: distraction from my (sometimes boring and often frustrating) real life, affirmation and validation, and connection. While Instagram or TikTok certainly provide distraction, using these apps passively is associated with less social connection, higher stress, and lower well-being.

The antidote? Finding affirmation, validation, and connection within real, in-person, not-online life. This is hard when you're a new parent and time is both nonexistent and somehow never-ending. *It's worth the effort, though.* Find other moms in your neighborhood (I highly recommend joining— and sucking at—a monthly mah-jongg group). Set up a standing call with a sister or friend who doesn't care if a tiny human screams in the background. Watch a thirty-minute TV show at the same time as a coworker and live text your reactions. Attend a meetup at the zoo or a support group at the hospital with new parents in your area. Go to the park and talk to a fellow parent, even for two minutes, about their experience raising their kid(s). Connection and encouragement in real life will always fill the bucket in a way that online connection cannot.

Yes, you came to this book for feeding advice and instead got a full chapter of nonexpert guidance on using social media less. You're welcome. In all seriousness, though, navigating the feelings that come with a disappointing feeding journey or a tough postpartum experience is only made harder by watching everyone else's situation online. Being mindful of how you use social media is a way to take care of yourself, and *you deserve to be cared for in this season (and always)*.

10

Why Is Pooping So Hard?

Before I had kids, I could have *never* imagined how much time I'd dedicate to talking about poop, looking at poop, worrying about poop, and cleaning up poop. It's gotta be the equivalent of days (maybe weeks?) at this point, even as my kids are older. The poop stress doesn't end in infancy, unfortunately! It is possible, however, to reduce this stress by understanding what's normal when it comes to infant bowel movements, which stool-related issues are worth a visit to the doctor, and what you can do to help promote healthy stools in your baby (and later, in your young child).

First, a Note on Straining

You've likely experienced this heartbreaking moment: Your

baby is straining, crying, and red in the face as they try to poop. As parents, it's natural to interpret these as signs that your baby is in pain. After all, if we were in pain while trying to poop, wouldn't it look just like that? This is a moment, however, to remember that babies are not simply tiny adults. What is obvious with our own experiences is not always correct when it comes to our baby's experiences! Many babies experience a harmless condition called *infant dyschezia*, which occurs when they struggle to coordinate the muscles needed to effectively bear down. We know that babies aren't born with good muscle control, and this includes the pelvic floor muscles that help push stool through and out of the digestive tract.

Crying and straining may look painful to the naked eye, but it is often the means a baby has to create the necessary intra-abdominal pressure to get the stool moving. These episodes of straining may last a few minutes, or even ten to twenty, and may occur every time your baby needs to have a bowel movement in the first weeks or months after birth. If the stool is soft when it appears (see discussion below on stool texture!), your baby may be experiencing infant dyschezia, not pain, as they try to poop.

Healthy, Normal Poops

When evaluating an infant's stool, focus on three features: color, texture, and frequency. These three can provide clues about whether an infant is tolerating their diet, whether they are digesting well, and whether there is a problem that should be evaluated.

Color: Normal infant poops are typically green, yellow, or brown. Sticky, black stool called *meconium* is normal in the few hours and days immediately after birth, but beyond that, black stool is a red flag. Most often—but not always!—breastfed babies experience yellow stools, which can be "seedy" with small undigested pieces of milk protein or milk fat. This is normal! Formula-fed babies often experience green stool, which occurs on account of the iron that formula is fortified with. Dark, hunter-green poop is not unusual for a formula-fed infant! Most babies, regardless of formula or breastfeeding, will change to having brown stool once solid foods are introduced, typically around the six-month mark. Black stools after the first few days of life, red stools (including those with fresh or old blood), and white stools are considered abnormal and should be evaluated by your child's doctor.

Texture: An infant's stool texture can vary, and many different textures are common. The most common, normal textures are soft (loose) and formed (with a pasty, peanut butter–like texture), although infants may also experience watery (liquidy) or hard (a formed, squishable shape, like Play-Doh) stools. Many factors influence an infant's stool texture, including whether an infant is breastfed or formula fed and how old the child is. Even the ingredients in a formula can impact stool consistency. For example, does the formula contain palm or palm olein oil, or does it have more casein protein than whey protein? Both palm or palm olein oil and more casein protein than whey protein can contribute to firmer stools! Does the formula contain partially hydrolyzed whey protein? Parents may notice looser stools. Both are fine.

There are, however, a few stool textures that parents should follow up on if they are seen consistently, and these are stools that are very loose and watery (clear and/ or frothy) for three or more diapers, or stools that are hard and pellet-like (think little rabbit poops).

Very watery or frothy stools may indicate a challenge with lactose (such as functional lactose overload in breastfed infants, or secondary lactose intolerance in formula-fed infants—particularly after a stomach bug). In either case, breastfeeding management or formula changes may be recommended. Hard, pellet-like stools that are also infrequent (like less than two bowel movements per week) may indicate constipation, and your pediatrician can likely suggest a variety of strategies to help soften the stool. These may include changing formulas, or, after about six months to one year of age, offering adequate water with meals and introducing *P* fruits like pears, prunes, or papaya.

Frequency: The range of "normal" bowel movement frequency in infants is incredibly wide, and this can be challenging for a new parent to wrap their head around! It can be perfectly healthy for an infant to poop five times a day, and it can be equally healthy for an infant to poop once every few days. Stool frequency alone matters much less than stool texture when evaluating for a problem. Infrequency is typically only a problem when combined with the hard, pellet-like stools described above, a history of large-diameter stools, a history of painful bowel movements, or other clinical indicators for at least one month. If the stool is soft when it appears, it's likely normal—even if it doesn't happen often.

Why do some babies poop more than others? Having a bowel movement depends on a variety of factors, and these will differ from baby to baby. These include diet, volume of formula or breast milk consumed, volume or type of solid foods consumed, proliferation of bacteria (good and/or bad) in the gut, and the effectiveness of pelvic floor muscles to move the stool along, among others. As an infant ages and they begin solids, stool frequency tends to settle into a one-to-three-times-per-day to every-other-day routine.

Baby Poop FAQs

My baby's poop has curds that look like pieces of undigested milk. Does this mean he's not digesting his bottles very well? Nope! Babies may have identifiable pieces of food (in this case, milk proteins or milk fat) in their stool just like adults. While there are a lot of mechanisms in place during digestion to break up food—milk, and later solids—some bits manage to make it through relatively intact. If your baby is gaining weight well and roughly maintaining their weight percentile, and they're not also experiencing diarrhea, they are very likely digesting and absorbing nutrients properly.

My baby's poop has mucus in it. Is this normal?

Mucus in stool is a tricky one to decipher—it can be completely normal, or it can be a sign of something underlying! Sometimes it occurs because a baby has congestion in the nose and throat that is swallowed, while other times visible mucus in the stool is an indication of irritation or infection in the gut. Some babies may experience irritation, and therefore mucus in the stool, due to excessive saliva being swallowed (like during teething). For others, excessive mucus in the stool can be a sign of an allergy or sensitivity to something they are consuming. If your baby has frequent or copious mucus in their stool, or has other symptoms that accompany the mucus like diarrhea, fever, or pain, discuss this with your child's pediatrician.

My baby had a stomach bug and now the diarrhea won't stop. What do I do?

This is a well-documented but rarely discussed phenomenon in parenting circles! After a GI bug, some children (and adults, for that matter), experience a form of temporary lactose intolerance called *secondary lactase deficiency*. This occurs when an illness, like gastroenteritis, damages the cells in the small intestine that produce lactase enzymes. These are the enzymes responsible for breaking down lactose, the milk sugar found in breast milk and other dairy-containing products like many infant formulas! If your child develops ongoing diarrhea after a stomach bug, talk to your pediatrician about whether to switch to a lactose-free formula if you are formula feeding. Although breast milk contains lactose,

the American Academy of Pediatrics recommends continuing breast milk in all cases for infants who are breastfed.
Generally, most infants with secondary lactase deficiency
will see no clinical advantage to moving to a low-lactose or
lactose-free formula unless the infant is considered at risk
(younger than three months or malnourished). Even so,
some parents may prefer to trial a lactose-free formula for
two to three weeks, after which their infant can resume a
lactose-based formula—often with a return to a more typical stool texture.

We started solids and now my baby is constipated. How can I help her be more comfortable?

It's amazing how quickly concerns about stool being too
loose switch to concerns about stool being too hard once
you introduce table food! Many babies experience firmer
stools once they're consuming solids. *P* fruits like pears and
prunes are often one of the first suggestions to soften stools,
though I find another easy solution is often overlooked:
Make sure you're offering water with your baby's meals!
Between six and twelve months, the American Academy of
Pediatrics recommends four to eight ounces of water a day
(beyond what's consumed via breast milk or infant formula).
Adequate, normal hydration can support softer, easier stools!

My baby is struggling with diaper rash. Is it related to what they're eating? Is there anything I can do to prevent it?

Diaper rash can be frustrating for parents and babies alike.
The key to preventing diaper rash is to keep their sensitive

skin protected from stool and urine, both of which can be irritating. That means changing diapers often and preventing the baby's skin from coming in contact with stool or urine as much as possible. Applying a barrier cream (either zinc-based or petrolatum-based) after cleaning your baby but before applying a fresh diaper can help! Some diaper rashes are caused by yeast, as the warm, moist environment inside a diaper is a perfect place for yeast to thrive. Allowing your baby to dry completely before applying cream and a fresh diaper is wise, and you can also allow them to go without pants for ten to fifteen minutes on a towel if they are not yet mobile. If you cannot seem to get the diaper rash to clear, consult with your pediatrician, as they may recommend an antifungal cream to treat it.

Quick Tip:
Check the Hands! Deciphering Hunger Cues

Did you know your baby's hands can give you a clue about whether they're hungry or full? It's true! And it's not complicated.

Tightly clenched hands can be a sign that your baby is hungry.

Loose, open hands (particularly during or after a feeding) can be a sign that your baby is full and content.

While not a foolproof method—sometimes babies' hands are clenched or loose for other reasons—this can be a helpful hint while you're learning how to decipher the rest of your baby's hunger and fullness cues. Try it next time! Watch your baby's hands throughout their next feeding. I'd be surprised if they didn't relax as your baby's tummy gets filled.

Mom Note
Unfortunately, Wearing Real Clothes Helps

I'll never forget waddling around Target the day I was discharged after my first birth (a C-section). Looking back, was it wise to attempt to walk around a retail store seventy-two hours after having my abdomen cut open? Definitely not. Zero out of five stars, I would not recommend, even with narcotic painkillers. But I did it anyway, for two reasons:

One, I wanted to feel *normal*. The experience of birth and early motherhood was so disorienting that I asked my husband to take me to Target so I could remember I was still a human in society like the rest of the humans wandering around there. It doesn't make sense, I know. But at the time, it felt important to me.

Two, I realized immediately after birth that none of my pre-pregnancy clothes were going to fit *for a while*, and the thought of putting back on my maternity clothes while not pregnant made me feel weird. Again, it doesn't make sense. I'm not arguing that my mental state was rational at that point—it most certainly wasn't. But having clothes that fit—that belonged on the bodies of "normal humans" and not specifically pregnant or postpartum ones—also felt important.

And you know what? Even if my thought process for why and how was questionable to start, the hypothesis was accurate: Wearing real clothes *was* important, and it dramatically helped my mental state.

Listen, I didn't want it to be true (if only for the sake of my comfort). It didn't make sense, logically, to wear anything other than pajamas postpartum if I was stuck in my house and spending half the day topless attached to a pump and the other half covered in spit-up. But when I made the commitment to put on real clothes—and we're talking athleisure, T-shirt dresses, and joggers here, not jeans—I started to see myself as *someone* rather than a collection of relevant body parts: breasts to feed my baby, hands to hold my baby, legs to walk and sway my baby, mouth to shush and hum for my baby.

Putting on real clothes helped me remember that I was a person who deserved to be taken care of—who deserved to be cared for—just like my baby. It provided a stepping stone to get out of the house (another crucial factor for my mental health discussed previously), because I was decently presentable if a whim struck me to go somewhere. It allowed me to be comfortable without feeling like a troll, which I'd argue is the inherent feeling of postpartum women everywhere if we're not intentional. It gave me one facet of my life that I could control even when so many others (feeding, sleeping, scheduling) felt out of my control.

While it was annoying—I had to fight many an urge of "What's the point?"—it was meaningful for me, and it may be for you, too. If you have the budget for it, get yourself something new and pretty that fits your current body, not the one you hope to have weeks, months, or years from now. Commit to wearing it once a week, and maybe throw a headband in your hair for good measure. See if it doesn't make you feel a bit more human and the world feel a bit more manageable. And heck, if it doesn't? Your pajamas are always there. My hunch, however, is that it will be worth it.

BABY AGE

3–6 Months

11

The Inconsistency
of Nipple Flows

Wouldn't it be great if there were more standardization when it comes to baby items? If every three-to-six-month onesie fit the same way, or if every brand had the same weight guidelines for their size-two diapers? This variability is fortunate for babies, who come in many different sizes and with many different needs, but it can be frustrating for parents who want to avoid the trial and error that comes with inconsistency among similar products.

There is another offender when it comes to this lack of standardization, and this one is crucial to know: There is *no consistency* in the rate of flow among "stages" or "levels" of nipples across brands.

What Is Nipple Flow Rate, and Why Does It Matter?

The size and shape of the hole in a silicone or latex bottle nipple determines the speed and volume of milk that can flow through it, as well as how much effort is required to withdraw the milk (i.e., how hard does a baby have to suck to be rewarded?). Nipple flow rates are designed to keep the flow of liquid through the nipple at a manageable level based on baby age. We don't want them to get overwhelmed by the flow, as this can lead to gagging, increased drooling, and coughing. Too fast a flow, or frantically feeding, often means a baby takes in excess air (while trying to catch their breath!), and this extra air can become painful trapped gas.

Most bottle brands package their bottles and sets with an included "slow flow," "stage one," or "level one" nipple. These are intended for newborns who need a very controlled flow of liquid as they learn how to feed effectively and efficiently. While some babies thrive using a slow flow nipple throughout their first year, bottle companies market (and parents tend to use) nipples with a faster rate of flow as their baby ages. These are typically called "medium flow," "stage two," or "level two" nipples, and later, "fast flow," "stage three," or "level three" nipples.

The challenge? The flow rate is *completely different* depending on the brand. A level three nipple in one brand may be as slow as a level two in another brand. A "slow flow" in one brand may be more similar to a preemie (sometimes called "stage zero" or "level P.") nipple in another. Additionally, the age ranges provided on the nipples' packaging are confusing. Dr. Brown's slow-flow, stage one nipple is advertised for ages zero months and older, while Philips Avent's Natural slow-flow nipple is advertised on the package for ages one month and older, while NUK has previously advertised their medium-flow Simply Natural nipple for one month and older. MAM's stage three nipple is advertised for four months and older, while Dr. Brown's shows six months and older on the packaging for their level three nipple. There is simply no consistency in labeling, just like there is no consistency in actual flow rate.

Instead of relying on number (stage or level), flow descriptor (slow, medium, medium-fast, fast), or age range, I encourage you to start with the nipple that came with the bottle and then look for signs that indicate the flow isn't working for your baby. Once you identify these signs, you can change to a different size accordingly—and ideally within the same brand for more accurate leveling up (or down) of flow rates.

Signs Your Baby's Nipple Flow Rate Is Too Fast

- Gagging, choking, or coughing while feeding

- Milk spilling out the sides of the mouth while feeding

- Gasping for air, or trouble coordinating sucking, swallowing, and breathing

- Gravity causes milk to drip from the nipple if you turn the bottle upside down; this is particularly not ideal if you have a baby less than six weeks old

Signs Your Baby's Nipple Flow Rate Is Too Slow

- You hear more sucks than swallows while feeding

- The baby is collapsing the top of the nipple while feeding because they are sucking so hard

- Your baby starts the feeding enthusiastically, but seems to get frustrated halfway through (spitting it out, turning red in the face, arching away from the bottle)

- Feeding takes longer than roughly twenty minutes, provided your baby is over the age of two months

Unfortunately, there is no real way to identify the correct nipple flow rate for your baby outside of trial and error. Keep in mind that if you go up a size, there may be a learning curve! It can sometimes take a day or two for a baby to figure out how to manage the faster flow. Employing paced feeding strategies (as discussed in chapter 8 on position while feeding) can help prevent overwhelm during the transition or when using a bottle nipple that is too fast, as this alone helps to reduce flow by counteracting gravity.

Quick Tip:
Batch, Please! The Gloriousness of Batching Formula

Here's the thing: I *love* a hack. I live for a tip or trick to reduce stress or time or money. I pride myself on finding efficiencies. Using a formula pitcher to batch a day's worth of formula might be my favorite hack ever.

Before we get into the what and how, let's review food safety rules for formula. Powdered formula that has been prepared *but not served to your baby* can be stored in the fridge for up to twenty-four hours. While this is true of individual bottles that are mixed and capped, it's also true for larger batches of formula that you can pour from as needed! Enter the formula mixing pitcher. This is one of my favorite pieces of feeding equipment on account of value given the amount of time it saves for the cost. These typically retail between ten and twenty dollars, and I certainly spent far more on far less effective tools and gadgets during my babies' early days.

A formula mixing pitcher allows a parent or caregiver to pour up to thirty-two ounces of water (tap, boiled, distilled, or purified—check with your pediatrician if you're unsure which to use), add in the appropriate number of scoops of powdered formula as indicated by the ratio of scoops to ounces of water on the back of your formula container, and mix using the included hand pump or battery-powered whisk (depending on the brand). Once mixed, the formula can be divided into individual bottles to quickly grab overnight or bring to day care, or can be kept in the pitcher—with the lid sealed and the whole thing stored in the refrigerator—to use as needed, just as long as the prepared formula is used within twenty-four hours of being prepped.

A few reasons why I loved using a formula pitcher:

1. I only had to do the math to count the scoops once per day. I don't know about you, but my counting skills are not ideal at two in the morning, and my brain was basically mush postpartum even during waking hours.

2. I could pour a conservative amount of milk from the pitcher into a bottle and then top up from the pitcher as needed if my baby still seemed hungry after (more on this in the next Quick Tip). This helped me reduce waste and keep my formula costs lower!

3. It made things very simple for a grandparent, nanny, or babysitter, as they simply had to pour

from the pitcher, and I didn't have to worry about them using the wrong water, adding too little or too much powder, or touching the formula container or scoop with dirty hands.

4. Preparing the formula at once and allowing it to sit in the fridge before use ensured that any foam or bubbles that formed when mixing had time to break up, thereby reducing the amount of air that my babies took in from their bottles during feeding.

5. It put formula prep on autopilot. I had a nightly routine to make the pitcher after dinner, and then I didn't have to worry about making formula for another twenty-four hours. The convenience was unmatched.

But Then the Formula Is Cold!

You're right—if you batch formula like this, it must be stored in the fridge. This means you either have to a) serve it cold or b) spend some additional time heating up a bottle after pouring the cold formula from the pitcher. My babies were willing to drink cold formula (and I knew there was no detriment in serving it that way), so that made it easy for us. If your

baby is picky about the temperature of their milk—
and some babies are—I've found placing the bottle
in a mug filled with hot water (from the sink is fine,
as long as it gets hot!) is a fast and efficient way to
take the chill off. Conventional bottle warmers can be
complicated, require frequent cleaning or descaling,
and take just as long. Keep a mug in your bedroom
or bathroom, fill it with warm water from the sink or
from a thermos, and pop the bottle in for a few minutes so that it warms gently without getting too hot.

A Pro Tip:
Switching from
Ready-to-Feed Formula

A formula mixing pitcher is also a great tool to use if
you're struggling to transition your baby from liquid
ready-to-feed formula to powdered formula. In my experience, allowing the formula to mix and then sit in the
fridge helped to improve the formula's texture (due to
the additional time for powder to dissolve and foam to
break up), making for a smoother liquid that was more
similar to what's found in ready-to-feed formula. Additionally, because ready-to-feed formula must be stored
in the fridge, offering your baby their pre-batched powder formula cold can make for an easy transition.

Mom Note
Resetting the Bar

Something I don't hear people talk about a lot? The mental and emotional impact of "failure" in parenthood, particularly if you've always been a high achiever. Many of us go through life with the understanding, and expectation, that if we prioritize and make the right calls and keep our noses to the grindstone, we will experience the outcomes we want. It can feel pretty straightforward:

- Studying hard leads to good grades.

- Networking leads to a job offer.

- Working out leads to muscle gain or weight loss.

- Exceeding expectations at work leads to a promotion or a raise.

And while this sort of cause and effect isn't always true or simple (and there are systemic privileges like sex or race that impact success), we're largely taught that working hard can get us the results we want.

But then we become parents, and this "if X, then Y" method of operating tends to go out the window.

Babies don't know that the books say they should nap for a certain length of time, or that the breastfeeding class taught that they should be able to latch without causing pain for mom, or that the safest way to sleep is on their backs alone in a crib. Often, to our dismay, they don't care. We—as parents—exist in a pressure cooker of shoulds and shouldn'ts, while babies couldn't care less. They do what they want, often with no regard for the effort we're expending trying to get them to do "what they should."

This reality was incredibly hard for me during my first experience postpartum. After all, *I was doing the right things!* Why wasn't it working?

To avoid driving myself crazy(-er), I had to deconstruct my definition of success and rebuild it. I needed to reset the bar for what a "successful" day, or even hour, looked like—one based on our reality and not an arbitrary metric some expert on the internet suggested was "best." I had to refocus my efforts *away* from trying to control outcomes I wasn't able to reliably, single-handedly control. It was hard.

Ultimately, having decided that I did not want to feel like a giant failure, I had to allow myself to believe that my success as a parent didn't hinge upon:

- My ability to breastfeed

- The number of ounces I was able to pump

- How well my baby slept

- How little my baby cried

- How quickly I could fit back into my pre-pregnancy clothes

- When (or whether) my baby met developmental milestones

- How well they grew on the growth curve

- Any other example of the myriad ways we judge ourselves as parents

Resetting the bar—for me—looked like acknowledging the effort, not the outcome, with a focus on how our home, and my body, felt. Did I eat when I was hungry today? That's success. Did I attend to my baby when she cried? That's success. Was I spending time learning more about this baby, and parenthood in general, so I could better serve her needs? That's success. Did she have clean clothes, clean bottles, and a dry diaper most of the day? That's success.

Resetting the bar is not the same as lowering standards.

It's about honoring smaller successes, because they matter as much as the big ones.

If you have a baby who can't or won't do "what they're supposed to do" according to the internet or the experts, and you're spinning your wheels and driving yourself bonkers trying to get them to do it anyway, it's okay to reset. It's okay to take a step back and evaluate whether you can change your definition of success.

Because when you refuse to hold something you can't fully control as the bar to meet, you also remove the ability to fail at it.

Resetting the bar for the statements listed above might look like:

- I'll breastfeed for as long as my baby and I are both thriving physically and otherwise.

- I will pump the amount my body allows me to pump, for as long as it's working for me physically and mentally.

- I will support my baby's sleep needs, and I will do what I can to prioritize my own sleep.

- If my baby cries, I will respond.

- I will honor my body's need for healing, and later, its need for movement.

- I will understand what developmental milestones are and when they should occur, and I will bring concerns to my baby's pediatrician if I have them.

- I will trust that my baby's body will grow at the rate it's supposed to grow.

It's much harder to "fail" at these things. They're significantly less binary in terms of "getting it right" or "getting it wrong." There is much more room for nuance—for the gray—when you refuse to treat parenthood as something you either win or lose based on rules someone else (who doesn't know you or your baby) has set.

If you find yourself feeling terrible about your parenting

all the time, it may make sense to reset the bar. Spend some time thinking through what success actually looks like for you and what smaller markers you can establish for getting there. If an expert says "X or Y is a must" and it isn't working for you, talk to your pediatrician about it. They tend to be much more reasonable than what you find on Instagram. You don't have to exist in a vacuum of all the ways you're "doing things wrong." If you feel like you are, step outside of it and measure success based on other things.

Please know I didn't work through this reframing challenge alone. Therapy was a crucial piece of this puzzle for me, as my therapist helped me sort through how I personally wanted to define success for me and my family. If you're stuck in negative thought patterns, please consider whether therapy could be a tool for you as well.

12

Supplementing and Combo Feeding

Breastfeeding doesn't have to be all or nothing. Many parents feed their baby with both breast milk and formula, a practice called *combination feeding, mixed feeding, supplementing with formula*, or simply *combo feeding*. For the sake of ease in this chapter, I will refer to any journey that includes nutrition from both breast milk and formula as *combo feeding*. Some may argue that supplementing and combo feeding are different, with *supplementing* being more limited in both volume of formula given and duration that formula is used, but I think that's splitting hairs. If you're feeding both formula and breast milk, you are combination feeding.

Why Combo Feed?

There are a variety of reasons why a family may need or choose to combination feed, and all are valid. Common reasons for combo feeding include:

- Insufficient milk supply

- Desire to reduce stress or pressure on mom as the only source of food for baby

- Desire to share feeding responsibilities (and joys!) with a partner

- Recommendation from a health care professional, sometimes due to a baby's poor weight gain

- Inability or disinterest in expressing breast milk using a pump upon returning to work

- Belief that this is the best way to feed a baby based on the family's circumstances or values

Any of these reasons (and a hundred others) are fine because you don't need any particular reason to combo feed or use formula with your baby!

Ways to Combo Feed

The *how* here often feels trickier than it is. *Combo feeding can look like whatever you want it (or need it) to look like.* Some families choose to alternate nursing sessions and formula bottles throughout the day. Others choose to nurse at night and send formula to day care. Others choose to offer one formula bottle a day to keep their baby acclimated to the taste and accepting of a bottle while breastfeeding the rest of the time. Still others combine breast milk and prepared formula in the same bottle to bring the volume up to a full serving. Some may nurse once a day for comfort or to provide antibodies during sick season and provide formula the rest of the time.

There's no right or wrong way to combo feed. There are considerations to think through that may inform how you do it (more on this later), but there's no "best practice" for doing this "right." However you want to do it, based on your needs and how much breast milk you can—or want—to provide *is fine.*

A Case Study: My Sister

My twin sister, Monica, is a combo feeding queen. She combo fed all three of her kids and found a system that worked well for her! She wanted to provide breast milk to her babies for their first six months of life while also getting them used to formula so she could transition to exclusively formula feeding after their half birthday. What worked for her was pumping four times a day, each roughly six hours apart: first thing in the morning, midday, last thing before bed, and one middle-of-the-night pump. Depending on how much her babies ate, this breast milk provided at least four full feedings' worth of breast milk per day, and she gave formula for the rest of the feedings. As her babies got older, she reduced to three pumping sessions a day and dropped the middle-of-the-night pump.

This worked for her for a few reasons:

1. Her goal was to continue to provide her babies with breast milk for a certain period of time, not a certain volume per day. By not getting hung up on how much she produced, anything she could pump and offer felt like a win.

2. Especially with her third baby, only pumping twice during her other kids' waking hours meant she was available for them the way she wanted to be.

3. She knew when she switched to exclusively formula feeding that her babies already liked the formula and didn't react to it.

4. She could share a lot of the feeding duties (making bottles and feeding) with her husband.

I'm not saying this is the perfect way to combo feed—only that it worked for her based on *her* goals and needs. If you want to combo feed, I'd encourage you to find a system that works for you and that you can feel good about (mentally and physically).

Considerations for Combo Feeding

Because breast milk production is thought to work on a supply and demand model, offering formula at some feeds without expressing or removing milk from your breasts simultaneously will likely result in reduced milk production. Unless you're exclusively breastfeeding your baby (and sometimes even then!), it can take a number of steps to establish and maintain a robust milk supply. If you choose to combo feed, be aware that you will need to either nurse or express breast milk at regular intervals throughout the day to continue to produce it. Work with a lactation consultant to identify a schedule for pumping, nursing, and formula feeding that is optimal for your milk supply and to meet your family's needs and your combo feeding goals.

There's also another challenge that comes with combo feeding, which is managing two sets of food safety rules at the same time. That's right! Formula food safety rules are different—and stricter—than breast milk food safety rules. Keeping track of these storage time frames for room temperature, in the fridge, and in the freezer (breast milk only!) can be tricky for new parents. If you plan to combination feed using bottles of formula and bottles of expressed breast milk, be sure to write when each was prepared or expressed and when each expires before leaving out at room temperature or storing in the fridge.

Transitioning from Combo Feeding to Exclusive Formula

If you've been a combo feeder and you're winding down your journey, know that the transition to full formula may not be difficult. I suggest trading out one breast milk feeding for a formula feeding a day and waiting around five days before dropping the next one, until you're transitioned over fully! Check out the tips in chapter 4 on how to dry up your milk safely as you transition.

Be aware that you may notice changes in your baby's digestion as you remove breast milk from their diet! Most notably, you may see changes in your baby's stool color (yellow to green) and frequency (more to less). These are common! If you notice your baby struggling to poop after switching to exclusively formula feeding, and you've given him or her a week to adjust, talk to your pediatrician.

13

Getting Ready for Day Care, a Nanny, or a Trustworthy Friend

The fourth trimester with a baby is the fastest and slowest time period known to humankind. Every day seems to last a lifetime, but somehow the weeks go by too fast and your baby changes too quickly. Author Jen Hatmaker once said having a baby is like spending five minutes underwater—five minutes is objectively not a long time, but it sure is when you're holding your breath! I found this analogy to be accurate for those early weeks of new parenthood, but before I knew it, I was twelve weeks postpartum and coming up for air. This also meant it was time for me to go back to work.

Whether you're returning to an in-office job, working from home with childcare, going back to school, or just needing some time away from your baby, you'll need to learn how to prep feedings for an outside caregiver. Here's what I suggest:

Hang Up Bottle Prep Guidelines: Whether you intend for a caregiver to prep a bottle or not, I always recommend printing the steps to make a bottle and hanging it on your fridge or elsewhere in your kitchen. Not only is this helpful for a future babysitter, it can also be a great reference when you're tired and your brain isn't functioning at full capacity when making bottles. Be sure these guidelines include washing hands before starting and the food safety rules for storage based on the type of milk (breast milk or formula) you're using.

Prep Bottles: The most foolproof way to ensure accurate and safe feedings when your baby is in someone else's care is to prepare bottles ahead of time, cap them, and store them in the fridge. Remember! Bottles that have been made but not yet offered to your baby are good for up to twenty-four hours in the refrigerator. In this case, make as many bottles as your baby will need while you're gone plus one extra in case, and leave instructions for warming the bottle—if your baby requires it warm—as well as guidelines about tossing any leftover formula within an hour of the beginning of the feeding.

Batch Formula for Pouring on Demand: If you're unsure how many bottles your baby may need and you have access to a fridge, consider making a batch of formula in a mixing pitcher and leaving instructions for your caregiver to pour a certain number of ounces before putting the collar and nipple on the bottle. Be sure to include guidance about washing hands first, keeping the pitcher in the fridge after use, and tossing any leftover formula in the bottle within an hour after beginning the feeding.

Preportion Water and Formula: If you won't have access to a refrigerator to prepare formula in advance, I suggest filling the number of bottles you need (plus one extra!) with water and then capping them. Then portion out the correct amount of formula for each bottle into clean, watertight containers. I like those that have different compartments for each feeding's worth of powder, so each compartment has the correct volume of powdered formula for the water volume in each bottle. Leave instructions for your caregiver to add one compartment of formula to one bottle when it's feeding time, and then swirl, stir, or shake to mix. Be sure to include guidance about washing hands first and tossing any leftover formula in the bottle within an hour after beginning the feeding.

Instructions for Post-Feeding: Provide clear guidance for what the caregiver should do after the feeding. This includes two parts: the documentation and the dirty bottle! First, the caregiver should note the start and end time of the feeding and how much your baby drank. Some parents choose to use an app that can be shared among caregivers (I like the Huckleberry app, personally), some day cares have a portal where they log details like this that parents can view online, and many others simply jot the information down on a piece of paper or send a quick text.

Second, let your caregiver know what to do with the bottle when the feeding is done. A formula bottle that has been offered and partially consumed should never be placed in the fridge to be used for another feeding. As such, parents may want the caregiver to dump any remaining formula, separate the bottle parts, and let them soak in warm soapy water or place them in the dishwasher. Others may want the bottles to sit in the sink without dumping out any remaining formula so that the parents can assess how much was consumed in their absence. In any case, giving caregivers clear guidance for what to do with bottles after feeding helps prevent an expired bottle from being reused later in the day.

Provide Space for Questions: Feeding rules evolve frequently based on changing AAP, FDA, and CDC guidelines. You should expect that some family members or babysitters will not be up-to-date on formula food safety rules and that you may even get pushback like, "We reused formula bottles from the fridge all day and you turned out fine!" I encourage you to presume positive intent—to assume they are coming from a place of helpfulness, and to respond with graciousness while being firm about your expectations. Leaving a phone number they can use to text questions, providing digestible reading material on updated guidelines, or having an honest conversation before their first time watching your baby can all help. Raising a baby is a group effort, and as much as possible, we want to keep those in our circle aligned while also keeping our baby safe.

Quick Tip:
The Top-Up Bottle

Babies aren't consistent eaters, especially in the first half of their first year. Sometimes they will eat four ounces at one o'clock in the afternoon, and the next day, they will only eat two and a half. Sometimes you prepare a large bottle and they only eat a quarter of it, while other times you prepare a smaller bottle and they act ravenous after they've drained it. It can be hard to estimate at any given feeding how much a baby will drink. This is frustrating because if you get it wrong, you can end up pouring formula (a.k.a. money) down the drain.

My favorite tip to reduce formula waste? Use a "top-up" bottle. Here's how it works:

1. Think about the maximum amount of formula your baby will drink in one feeding, even if they only drink that much occasionally. For this example, let's say it's six ounces.

2. Think about the minimum amount of formula your baby will *always* eat in one feeding. Let's say it's four ounces.

3. Subtract the minimum volume from the maximum. In this case, that's a two-ounce differential.

4. Math is over! Now it's time for formula prep: Make a bottle with the *maximum* number of ounces. In this case, six ounces!

5. Grab a second, clean bottle.

6. Pour the *differential* number from the first bottle into the second bottle. In this example, you'd end up with four ounces in the first bottle, because you've poured the extra two ounces of it into the second bottle.

7. Cap the second bottle, which is your top-up bottle.

When your baby's hungry, offer the first bottle. If they drink all the milk and are still acting hungry, add another half ounce or ounce from the top-up bottle. Continue this until they're full. If they don't drink the original bottle or they finish it and seem satisfied, you're done and the top-up bottle goes into the fridge for the next feeding, and you've saved two ounces from going down the drain (because remember, if that extra two ounces had been in the first bottle, you'd have to toss it if your baby didn't consume it within an hour).

This may feel complicated the first time you do it, but it quickly becomes second nature. It's simply a way to get ahead of the inconsistency in volume that babies eat by offering them more if they actively demonstrate they want more versus presuming from the start that they will. Having the extra easily on hand but not in the bottle they're currently drinking means you can save it in the fridge if they don't want it. A win all around!

Mom Note
It's Okay to Not Want to Leave Your Baby

My second baby was—and is—the sweetest boy I've ever known. He's snuggly, he's giggly, he's happy to be here. From the first moment I saw him, I felt an immense attachment to him. This was a totally different experience from our firstborn, and I can't tell you how or why things were different, but they were. I suddenly understood why everyone said having a baby was the best. Because *he* was the best. He was my sweet little buddy and still is. And because of this? I was selfish with him. (Perhaps *selfish* isn't the right word, as I'm not sure you can really be selfish with your own baby. I'm sure you get the gist.)

Looking back, I worked really, really hard for him. It took an immense amount of courage, after having such severe postpartum depression with my first, to try for another baby. I was in therapy during the pregnancy. I stayed on my mental health medication. He brought me lots of nausea and vomiting, a kidney stone at thirteen weeks, a gestational diabetes diagnosis and four blood sticks a day for months, tons of extra appointments with maternal-fetal medicine, and a repeat C-section. The journey to him was fraught on all levels, and when he arrived, he was *mine*. For a long time, I wasn't keen on letting others have a turn with him.

It's okay if you don't want to leave your baby with someone else. This is a totally normal (some might say biological) response.

If you're able to keep your baby with you, and that feels like the best option, go for it! Don't feel pressured to "socialize" your baby by introducing them to other people if you don't want to. That will come with time. These feelings—that you need and deserve more time with your baby before you start sharing—are completely normal.

I do, however, want to speak to two specific scenarios that are inextricable from this conversation, as sometimes whether or not you leave your baby doesn't feel like much of a choice at all.

Postpartum anxiety: It is common for parents to feel trepidation about someone else watching their baby—even someone well qualified! After all, you know your baby best, and your baby knows (and trusts) you most. They recognize your voice and smell, and they lean on you to meet their needs and offer them comfort. It's reasonable to feel nervous about whether someone else will do things the right way and to worry about whether your baby will be safe and comfortable in your absence.

Some parents experience a very significant level of anxiety beyond these typical concerns. Clinical postpartum anxiety can cause parents tremendous distress when only *thinking* about spending time away from their baby. Signs and symptoms of postpartum anxiety (according to the Cleveland Clinic) can include:

- Increased heart rate or heart palpitations

- Difficulty sleeping, even when exhausted (often for fear of something bad happening to your baby if/ while you sleep)

- Frequent thoughts of harm or danger regarding you or your baby that others may consider irrational

- Worry that feels unmanageable, and/or like it will never go away

If you are experiencing anxiety that is disruptive to your functioning or comes with intrusive thoughts, please discuss this with your doctor. You deserve to enjoy your postpartum period! You can also visit Postpartum Support International (PSI) at www.postpartum.net or call 1-800-944-4773 for toll-free support from the PSI Helpline.

Return to work: I think we can all agree that the United States has an abysmal parental leave policy (a.k.a. no paid leave policy on the federal level, and even unpaid leave covered by the Family and Medical Leave Act, or FMLA, is not guaranteed in certain circumstances). Some parents return to work within a few days or weeks, others are able to take up to twelve weeks (paid or unpaid), while others may have more time (paid or unpaid) through their employer or state. Very few Americans take off twelve to eighteen months for parental leave, which is offered in other countries like Canada, the UK, and Australia.

Many of us go back to work before we feel physically, mentally, and/or emotionally ready, and this often requires us to leave our babies in the care of someone else even if we don't want to. I don't have an answer other than to say: I'm with you. It's really hard. I wish things were different. I wish you had more time.

A comfort to me, even now as a working mom with a number of years under my belt, is a phrase from Jennifer Walker, RN, BSN, of Moms on Call—one of my favorite resources for infant feeding and sleep guidance—who says, "We may not always be there, but they know we're always *theirs*." Even ten years into my parenting journey, the sentiment makes me tear up. Our babies know us. They are attached to us. Even if we spend eight or ten or twenty-four hours away from them, they know they are ours and we are theirs.

Your absence won't damage your bond, and when you're home, it's okay to be selfish with that baby. Let them nap on you (while you're awake!), don't feel pressured to pass them to

Grandma, and do tummy time on your chest so you're facing each other. The time apart can make the time together sweeter, even if we wouldn't choose the time apart if we had the choice.

Mom Note
It's Okay to Want to Leave Your Baby

When my first baby was five weeks old, my husband and I went away for a weekend. *Without her.* My mother-in-law came into town, and we left our daughter what little pumped milk I'd collected, plus some formula, and we flew to the beach. My husband surprised me with the trip, as I would've undoubtedly told him no if he'd asked before booking the flight. Not because I didn't want the break but because I didn't feel like I deserved one. He, however, could see how quickly I was falling into a deep hole of postpartum depression, so he did the only thing he could think to do—he brought me to the place I'd always been happiest.

Did getting two full nights of sleep and sitting in the sun make everything better? Not by a mile, but it did help me remember that I was still a person outside of being a mom. It also gave us the time and space to make a game plan for managing my PPD when we returned, which we decided meant quitting the pump, starting therapy, increasing the dosage on my mental health medication, and splitting the night shift so we each got a few hours of guaranteed consolidated sleep every night.

That weekend away was pivotal for me, and I didn't tell

anyone about it *for years*. I was embarrassed and ashamed. I thought, *What kind of mom leaves her baby when she's not even two months old?* and *What kind of mom* wants *to leave her brand-new baby?* I thought people would judge. When I started to tell this story on the Formula Mom Instagram page, people *did* judge. But looking back, nearly ten years later? Getting away for forty-eight hours was the best thing we could've done for our family. I don't regret it for a second.

Now, I am not suggesting that everyone leave their baby for a weekend at only a few weeks old. With our second baby, we didn't spend a night away from him for months, and that worked well for us in that season. But if you want some time off or feel like you need some time off, and you have the support and means to take it? *Take the time away.* Whether it's thirty minutes, three hours, or three days, your baby isn't going to be less bonded or irreparably traumatized by your absence while you collect yourself.

I know our current societal narrative doesn't support this idea. Social media will try to tell you that even putting your baby down for a nap in their room by themselves is harmful and that babies need to be with their mothers 24-7 to promote healthy attachment. However, healthy attachment is influenced by a number of factors, and it is strongly formed when the attachment figure provides stability and safety in moments of stress. The state of parents' health and "the degree of the mother's fulfillment of her responsibilities for her child (interest, love, education, health, and financial resources)" also influence attachment!

Constant parental companionship for a baby wasn't true of

prior generations, though a certain segment of people online like to paint a picture of homesteading families with an infant on their hip while homeschooling older children before co-sleeping—spending every minute together as a nuclear family.

In reality, working parents spend *more* time with their children now than stay-at-home parents did in generations past, and centuries ago, families often lived in multigenerational communities where babies were cared for by a variety of family members, not just their parents. It has never been normal (or expected!) for a baby to spend every waking—and sleeping—moment with their mom. And wouldn't you know, babies learned to walk and talk and eat and sleep all the same in decades past.

Hear me say this: There is nothing wrong with you if you want an occasional break from your baby. It doesn't mean you don't love them. It doesn't mean you suck as a mother or that some supposedly inherent maternal instinct is broken within you. It doesn't mean you're replaceable and that anyone else can step in and do your job. (These are all real thoughts I had—maybe you don't, and in that case, I'm happy for you!) All it means is that you're human, because *all humans need and desire rest.*

If you want to leave your baby and have the means to do so (money for a babysitter, a trusted friend, a helpful mother-in-law, a kind neighbor), take some time for yourself. Do whatever will make you feel like you again, and don't judge yourself for it. Take a walk in the park, sit in the sun, wander leisurely around the mall, get your hair done, drive through Taco Bell and eat in the car while scrolling TikTok (my preferred break of choice, even now). With our daughter, we took two full days away. With our son, I had a babysitter come for two hours each week until I went back to work. Both were needed, and both helped me manage the postpartum season a bit better.

No one prepares you for how relentless parenting is. It's okay to take a break, particularly if that break will help you come back to the demands of parenting with renewed energy.

If you want a break—and can make it happen—take it.

14

Traveling with Formula

It's time to hit the road, baby! Whether it's your first trip with your first baby or you simply need a refresher with a new little one, there is a lot to consider before traveling with your formula-fed baby. While we'll focus on plane and car trips, the advice provided for airline travel is also applicable for travel by train and boat.

But First, What Type of Formula?

We discussed in chapter 2 that formula comes in a variety of formats, including liquid ready-to-feed, liquid concentrate, and powdered varieties. Certain parents view certain formats as more convenient for travel than others. Some prefer to travel with powdered formula, even if they use ready-to-feed at home, because they can make each bottle fresh without the refrigeration required for larger, thirty-two-ounce bottles of ready-to-feed formula once opened. On the other hand, some parents who use powdered formula at home prefer to use liquid ready-to-feed formula when traveling (in two-ounce or eight-ounce bottles that can be used in one sitting) because they don't want to mess with water and the risk of spilling powder on a bumpy flight.

Both options are fine! I would caution you, however, *not to assume* that if your baby takes a certain brand or type of formula in one format they'll easily accept it in another. Liquid ready-to-feed formulas contain certain ingredients—like stabilizers and emulsifiers to keep them from separating—that powdered formulas do not. Additionally, the texture of powdered formula versus ready-to-feed liquid formula is different! If you plan to use a different formula format while traveling from what you typically use at home, do a trial run or two before your trip to ensure your baby accepts the new format.

Plane Travel

Packing for a flight with a formula-fed baby can be a logistical challenge. Here's what I recommend:

- **Pack more bottles than you'll need:** Travel days are known to upend even the most steadfast feeding and sleeping schedules. Your baby may be distracted by the excitement around them and drink less than usual; they may be anxious and want to eat more than usual, as sucking is known to help soothe; or unexpected delays may mean travel lasts longer than you anticipated. I'd suggest bringing one and a half to two times the number of bottles you would normally need for the time period you'll be in transit, as it's much better to have more than you need than to need more than you have!

- **Pack more formula than you'll need:** Same thinking applies here—it's better to be prepared than to find yourself lacking formula when your baby is hungry while traveling. If possible, it's a great idea to portion your powder (if that's what you're using) into your baby's serving size ahead of time to minimize the need to count, level, and dump scoops while in the air. A portable formula dispenser works great for this!

  Here's a confession: I didn't pack enough formula during a trip to Sint Maarten when my oldest was six months old, and I rate the experience zero out of ten stars. It was so stressful! Bring twice what you think you'll need for the trip. You have a few options for how to transport formula, and these include bringing as much as possible in your carry-on luggage, packing your formula in a checked bag and praying your bag doesn't get lost (consider placing an AirTag tracker in it!), or researching your destination before you leave to learn what type of formula is available and how you might access it from wherever you're staying. I personally suggest carrying on as much formula as you can—after my mishap in the Caribbean, I've been known to pack a full hard-shell suitcase with just formula in it. We do what we have to do!

While manufacturers recommend keeping formula in its original container to reduce risk of bacteria introduction, some families may choose to transition their formula into a more space-friendly container for trips. My sister prefers to transfer her formula into clean gallon-size zip-top plastic bags (along with the scoop!) and then double-bag it to prevent tears or spills. This allows the formula to be packed flat. While I can't formally recommend this since these bags are not sterile, if your baby was full-term and is not immunocompromised, you can assess—ideally with input from your pediatrician— whether the space-saving is worth the risk inherent in the transfer.

- **Know what's allowed:** The Transportation Security Administration, or TSA, provides guidance on traveling with breast milk, formula, baby food, and more. These are considered "medically necessary liquids" and are not subject to the 3.4-ounce rule that other liquids are. It is recommended to let your TSA officer(s) know you are traveling with formula and to remove your formula or other liquid foods from your carry-on bags before screening. Build in extra time to get through security as, in my experience, TSA will want to swab your formula container and/or pat it (or you) down. While the TSA website does not explicitly state that water to be used for mixing formula is allowed in excess of 3.4 ounces, some parents are able to get it through. I recommend buying water on the other side of security.

- **Get water (and keep it safe):** Always use water from a safe source when preparing your baby's formula, whether tap water or bottled water. If you choose to purchase bottled water at the airport, I recommend labeling your baby's water so it doesn't accidentally become someone else's drink—we don't want our germy mouths on our baby's water source! Feel free to label your own as well. It can also be helpful to pour your baby's water into their bottles before you get on the plane—and then cap them—so you don't risk water on your lap when trying to pour midair.

    Need the water to be boiled? Since it's typically not possible to boil water to sterilize it (or the formula) while traveling, liquid ready-to-feed formula is recommended for those who need a sterile product. Choose smaller volumes, like two-ounce or eight-ounce bottles or cartons, so any extra can be tossed (freeing you from the need to keep it cold for the next feeding).

- **Consider bringing a portable bottle warmer:** If your baby is picky about their bottle temperature, consider investing in a portable warmer. There are a handful of rechargeable, battery-operated warmers that are perfect for travel or on the go! Check with your preferred brand to ensure the product is TSA-approved for carry-on or checked luggage.

- **Identify a bag for dirty bottles:** Once your baby is happily fed, you'll need somewhere to store their used bottles! I recommend bringing an empty gallon-size zip-top bag or a plastic grocery bag where you can place bottle parts after the bottle has been dumped and rinsed. Label it so it's clear the bag is for bottles that are dirty! These will need to be washed eventually, of course, but segregating them into a "dirty bag" reduces the likelihood that an hours-old bottle gets picked up from the pocket of the diaper bag and accidentally reused.

- **Bring dish soap and a small brush:** It's not ideal to wash bottles in a hotel bathroom sink. We don't really want our bottles chilling in the sink with all of our mouth germs from brushing our teeth! But if you have some dish soap and a small bottle brush, it's doable, and your plastic bag is going to come in handy again. Take your dirty bottle parts out and put them on the counter, rinse out the bag, and fill it halfway with warm, soapy water. Put your bottle parts back in, seal or clamp off the top of the bag, and slosh those bottles around! We want that warm soapy water to wash all the pieces.

You can set the bag down in the basin of the sink to take each piece out, scrub with the brush, and then rinse. Washed and rinsed bottle pieces can be placed on a clean, dry hand towel to air-dry. Once you're done, rinse the soapy water from the bag, hang it to dry, and use it the next time you need to clean your bottles! I recommend having a few bags (two to five) in case any of them get split or damaged.

- **Pack a sterilizer microwave bag:** If the place where you're staying has a microwave, consider purchasing and bringing sterilizer bags with you. These are multiuse! Follow the instructions to place bottle parts in the bag, add water, and place in a microwave for the indicated number of seconds. The heat plus water creates steam, which kills bacteria. This can provide extra assurance if you're not convinced your bathroom sink cleaning attempt is as thorough as you'd like.

- **Feed on takeoff and landing:** Air travel can be hard on babies, and one reason is they don't know how to intentionally equalize—or "pop"—their ears. They also have relatively narrow tubes that connect the middle ear to the back of the throat (called *eustachian tubes*), whose role is to help equalize air pressure. We know how uncomfortable it is to have a "clogged" ear from a plane trip, and we don't want that for our babies! Feeding them during takeoff and landing can help, as the motion of the jaw when sucking and swallowing promotes equalization.

- **Adopt an "it's fine" attitude:** Traveling with a baby can be a dumpster fire. I once had to board a plane with a baby in nothing but a diaper because she'd had a massive diaper blowout up the back of her onesie and I didn't have time to change her before our connection—that onesie went straight into the trash on the way to the gate! Going into your trip prepared, but with low expectations, tends to make travel easier. Even if things go sideways—your baby doesn't nap, the formula spills, they scream the entire plane ride and your mom has to walk up and down the aisle bouncing them while you silently cry from frustration in your seat (i.e., me on the way back from that same Sint Maarten trip)—it's fine. Things will almost certainly be better the next day. Get through the travel however you have to, pat yourself on the back for making it, and let your normal expectations go.

Car Travel

Taking a road trip with a baby tends to be easier than a plane ride—they're strapped into a car seat the whole time, you can stop when you want, and if you need more of something, a grocery store is likely to be a few exits away. While some of the advice for car travel is the same as for plane travel (see the following above: Pack more bottles and formula than you think you'll need, bring a bag for dirty bottles, consider a bottle warmer and microwave sterilizer bags if desired, and don't forget soap and a bottle brush!), there are a few unique considerations to be aware of.

- **Bring enough water:** Gallons of water are great for car travel! Keep them at room temperature and make sure they stay capped when not in use. If you know you'll have access to water for formula when you arrive, you can instead pour any water you may need into your baby's bottles ahead of time, and stop along the way if you happen to run out.

- **Prep ahead or make fresh:** As a reminder from chapter 7, a prepared but unserved bottle is good for up to two hours at room temperature or up to twenty-four hours in the fridge. Depending on the length of your drive, you may choose to make bottles fresh as you need them (pour your preportioned powder into the preportioned water!). If you'd like to make bottles more than two hours ahead, you'll need to ensure they stay at refrigerator temperature—ideally between 35 and 40 degrees Fahrenheit. If you're not certain that your cooler and ice packs can maintain this temperature long-term, it's better to make each bottle fresh!

- **Stop to feed:** While it can be tempting to feed your baby their bottle while they're strapped into their car seat while you're moving (thus reducing the length of the trip), it's recommended to stop and bring your baby into your arms for each bottle feeding. Not only is the break good for them (it's recommended to stop to rest and stretch every two hours on a road trip anyway), it also reduces the likelihood that your baby chokes, aspirates, or allows liquid in the back of their mouth to drain into the eustachian tubes—this can increase risk of ear infections. Additionally, bottles can become dangerous projectiles in the case of a crash. Best practice is to stop and attend to your baby when they're hungry versus journeying on.

The Juice Is (Likely) Worth the Squeeze

Traveling with a baby requires a lot of logistical planning and can be an exercise in letting go of control—particularly with schedules. Even so, I've almost always found the effort to be worth it. Seeing new places, making new memories, introducing your kid(s) to different experiences and cultures—even if they won't remember them—can be a good reward for the stress of travel. While you may come back from your vacation needing a vacation (as a family friend once said, "A vacation with kids isn't a vacation but a relocation"), I hope the memories you make will have been worth it.

15

Introducing a Schedule

Before we start this chapter, I need you to know this: *You do not need to get your baby on a schedule.* If you aren't bringing your baby to day care or to a sitter who watches other infants, you can be as loosey-goosey as you want. You can follow your baby's lead and let them sleep when they're tired and eat when they're hungry and play when they want to play. This is totally fine! Many families operate this way, and it works for them.

However, if you'd like to implement a schedule (or need to), it's not as scary of an endeavor as you may think. In my experience, a schedule can help reduce stress and anxiety for the caregiver by eliminating *What do I do next?* thoughts throughout the day. Additionally, it can help parents or caregivers anticipate their baby's needs, getting ahead of hunger or tiredness before their baby becomes fussy. Lastly, having a schedule provides a measure of certainty when making plans with family members, playdates, or time away from the baby. If you know when they will eat or sleep, making decisions about out-of-the-house events becomes easier.

A few principles to ground us before we dig into the *how* of infant schedules:

- I don't recommend trying to implement a schedule under eight to twelve weeks of age (or adjusted age for premature babies). Before this, it's recommended to feed your baby on demand. Please discuss with your pediatrician before introducing a schedule, as they may have benchmarks (such as a certain weight or age) they recommend before moving away from a feed-on-demand model.

- With infants, a schedule provides a *framework*, not an instruction manual. As I've referenced in prior chapters, babies don't always do what we want! A schedule exists to loosely structure the day with a baby, but even so, we must adopt a spirit of flexibility to accommodate for changing needs.

- If your baby is hungry, feed them! Again, a schedule is simply a guide. We don't want to listen to the schedule more than we listen to our baby. While I will share sample schedules in this chapter, do not put off feeding your baby if they're hungry but it's not yet "time." Feeding gets priority!

- You know that old adage "Don't wake a sleeping baby"? I disagree. Often, keeping a schedule, even if that means waking a baby during the day to feed, can contribute to longer stretches of sleep at night. And listen, I know it's painful. I know they look so peaceful and content with their (envy-inducing) eyelashes fanned across their cheeks. I know you want to spend another fifteen minutes on your phone in blissful silence. *I know.* But if you want your baby to be on a consistent schedule, you will sometimes have to wake them up.

- You can adjust the schedule based on your needs. The schedules you'll see below show a 7:30 a.m. wake time and a 7:30 p.m. bedtime because that's what worked for our family. You can shift this schedule by any measure of time so long as the entire schedule shifts and not just the wake time or the bedtime.

The Priority When Scheduling

I always recommend prioritizing a certain number of feedings per day, based on your baby's age, and then working in naps around it. Why is this important? Because if your baby doesn't get sufficient calories during the day, they will need to consume those missing calories at night. Waking at night to eat is normal, especially in early infancy! But as your baby gets older, an easy way to promote overnight sleep is to ensure that sufficient, full feedings take place during the day. As such, the main markers for the schedules below are feeding times, targeting five to eight feedings a day in the early months, with space for naps and play in between.

A Consistent Wake Time

A key part of getting your baby on a schedule is to establish a consistent wake time every morning. For our family, this was 7:30 a.m. This meant no matter what happened overnight, we woke our baby for the day at 7:30 a.m.—even if they had just been up to eat at 6:00 a.m. or 6:30 a.m. Again, *this is painful*, especially when you are exhausted as a parent. This is short-term pain for long-term gain, however, and you'll reap the benefits sooner than you think.

Sample Schedule: Three to Six Months

The three-to-six-months schedule below is ideal for babies who have not yet started solids and whose parents want to promote sleeping through the night. While I can offer no guarantees, this schedule allowed both of our kids to sleep through the night (defined as ten or more hours of uninterrupted sleep) by five months of age without any formal sleep training. The key at this age is to try to never go more than three hours between feedings. Often parents want to *extend* the time between feedings, and I caution you not to! Keeping the interval between feedings at three hours or less ensures your baby will have five or six feedings during waking hours.

The amount of formula your baby takes in each day in months three to six may vary. In general, by six months of age, a baby will usually drink about six to eight ounces at four or five feedings a day—and, on average, no more than about thirty-two ounces of formula in twenty-four hours. If your baby takes more or less, that may be fine! Check with your pediatrician, as many are less concerned about total daily volume intake as long as the baby's growth curve percentile remains relatively consistent.

Here's what I suggest for babies three to six months old:

- 7:30 a.m.: Wake and feed

- 10:30 a.m.: Feed

- 1:30 p.m.: Feed

- 4:30 p.m.: Feed

- 7:30 p.m.: Feed and bedtime

- (10:30 p.m.: Dream feed—see the Quick Tip next)

Sample Schedule: Six to Nine Months

While it can feel tempting to extend the amount of time between feedings or start dropping bottle feedings or nursing sessions in favor of solids at this point, I again encourage you not to. At this stage, solids provide exposure to different tastes and textures and the opportunity for your baby to develop their oral motor skills, and the nutrition complements what is found in formula or breast milk. But most of the nutrition they get should still come from formula or breast milk, as much of the food you serve will end up in their hair and on the floor anyway during this season! As such, I recommend continuing to prioritize five feedings a day, at the same three-hour interval, and adding meals *on top of these feedings* versus instead of them.

If a baby is consuming up to thirty-two ounces of breast milk or formula per day in months six through nine, with five feedings a day, each of these feedings will likely be between six and seven ounces. If your baby takes more or less, that may be fine! Check with your pediatrician, as many are less concerned about total daily volume intake as long as the growth curve percentile remains relatively consistent.

Here's what I suggest for babies six to nine months old:

- 7:30 a.m.: Wake and feed

- *(Optional: Breakfast solids with family)*

- 10:30 a.m.: Feed

- 1:30 p.m.: Feed

- 4:30 p.m.: Feed

- *Dinner solids with family*

- 7:30 p.m.: Feed and bedtime

Sample Schedule: Nine to Twelve Months

Your baby's first birthday is growing nearer, and this means thinking about the switch from milk as the primary source of nutrition to food as primary. As such, now is when you will begin extending the interval between feedings and begin to replace bottle feedings with meals or snacks. Note: I suggest one "solids" meal a day from six to seven months, two "solids" meals a day from eight to ten months, and three "solids" meals a day from eleven months forward. Commonly, babies consume six to eight ounces of breast milk or formula three or four times a day during the nine-to-twelve-month age range.

As you gradually introduce more solids, you may find that the amount of formula or breast milk your baby consumes decreases. This is a natural part of the transition to solids! Remember, your baby's feeding needs are unique and can vary. If your baby takes more one day and less another, that may be fine. Check with your pediatrician, as many remain less concerned about total daily volume intake as long as the growth curve percentile remains relatively consistent.

Here's what I suggest for babies nine to twelve months old:

- 7:30 a.m.: Wake and feed (bottle)

- *Breakfast solids with family*

- 10:30 a.m.: Snack

- *Lunch solids with family*

- 1:30 p.m.: Feed (bottle)

- 4:30 p.m.: Feed (bottle)

- *Dinner solids with family*

- 7:30 p.m.: Feed (bottle)

A Reminder!

It may take your baby (and you) a few days to acclimate to a schedule. It may be a mess for the first few days, and that's to be expected. I encourage you to stick with it if a schedule is important to you! On the flip side, some families may discover that these sorts of prescriptive schedules don't work for them. If you try it and it doesn't work for you (or your baby), that's okay! It doesn't mean there is something wrong with you or wrong with your little one—some babies are more amenable to structure than others.

Additionally, a set schedule may *increase* worrying in some parents, as they wonder what to do if their baby misses a feeding time or doesn't eat as much as they "should." If attempting a schedule makes you feel worse, throw the whole thing away! The best part of parenting is that you get to decide what works for you and for your family. You have agency to say yes or no to systems or methods that others suggest, and just because someone else loves something doesn't mean you have to (or that you're a failure if you don't).

My wish for you is to find the rhythms that work for your family and the unique needs contained therein. Schedule or no schedule, that's what is most important.

Quick Tip:
The Dream Feed

Is there anything better than snuggling with a warm, squishy, sleepy baby? I'm not sure there is—they're like nature's weighted blanket. Holding my sleepy babies during the *dream feed* every night was one of my very favorite parts of their infancy, and it might be your favorite, too!

What Is a Dream Feed?

A dream feed is a breast or bottle feeding that takes place when your baby is partially or fully asleep, with the goal of providing parents (yes, you!) with longer stretches of time to sleep. When I refer to the dream feed, I'm specifically referencing a feeding that takes place roughly three hours after the baby's bedtime but before the parent goes to bed. For us, this looked like a 7:30 p.m. baby bedtime, a 10:30 p.m. dream feed, and then an 11:00 p.m. parent bedtime.

The mechanics are as simple as it sounds. When it's time for the dream feed, you pick your baby up from their crib or bassinet, offer them a bottle to drink (which could be the same number of ounces you offer during the day), burp them, and then place them back down to sleep. Because sucking is a reflex for babies, some will drink the bottle without fully waking up, and this is okay! You don't have to change their diaper before or after this feeding unless they have had a bowel movement, as this tends to wake them up. Simply lift them into your arms, feed them, and put them back to bed.

Why, Though?

In theory, a dream feed helps your baby sleep longer and maximizes the chance that you, as the parent, get a few hours of consolidated sleep. There are two ideas as to why a dream feed might help: First, filling up your baby's stomach one more time may help reduce the likelihood that your baby will be up to eat in the first few hours of your night. Second, babies often have their longest stretch of sleep earlier in the night. Some parents report that by gently interrupting their baby's sleep via a dream feed, they can effectively "reset the clock" to push that longest stretch of sleep into the same window as their parental sleep. For example, if a baby is capable of sleeping for five straight hours, it's ideal for that five-hour stretch to coincide with the time the parent is also sleeping (for example, 11:00 p.m.–4:00 a.m. versus 7:00 p.m.–12:00 a.m.).

Age Range

I recommend the dream feed be introduced between three and six months. At this age, babies usually weigh enough to sleep through the night (roughly twelve or more pounds), and parents may be eager to implement a plan to promote good sleep. After solids are started at around six months of age, you may find that your baby doesn't need a dream feed, especially if they are consuming enough calories during waking hours. While dropping the dream feed can feel scary ("What if my baby starts waking up again to eat at night?"), around six months, babies tend to develop regular sleep schedules, and they may sleep straight through without it.

For Babies Who Spit Up

For babies with reflux, you may need to work on a burp and keep them upright for some time (fifteen minutes or more) after the dream feed before putting them back down. This can help reduce the risk that their feeding will come back up!

Not Working for You?

Like everything else, not all strategies work for all babies. Some babies are easily awoken, and attempting a dream feed can throw them into a full wake cycle—they can be difficult to get back to sleep for forty-five to sixty minutes after. If this is the case for you, scrap the dream feed! Take what works for you and dump what doesn't. It may be worth trying a few times to ensure it wasn't a fluke, but if the dream feed consistently *reduces* the likelihood of good sleep (for baby or you!), it's not worth doing. In this case, be sure to prioritize feedings during waking hours to get enough nutrition in during the day before your baby's bedtime.

16

To Feed or Not to Feed? Dealing with Night Wakings

It's three o'clock in the morning, and you wake to the sound of your baby fussing. You drag yourself out of bed, rub your eyes, and approach the crib wondering when you will ever get a full, uninterrupted night's sleep again. You reach in to pick your baby up, assuming they are hungry, but then you *stop* because you hear my voice in your head saying:

They might not be hungry! Let's wait a minute!

Okay, so maybe that won't happen, but the point remains: As parents, we often assume our babies are hungry at night when they are crying. In the early weeks of infancy, this tends to be the case! Sometimes, though, this assumption is wrong, and starting the habit of feeding a baby at night who isn't actually hungry can create an endless loop of wakings night after night. We don't want this!

If you know your baby is getting sufficient calories during the day as a result of feeding well during daytime hours, regular wet and dirty diapers, and consistent, appropriate growth, I recommend *not* offering a bottle at night *until other strategies have been tried*. Note: I am not now (or ever) saying to ignore a hungry baby. Instead, I'm suggesting you take a minute or two to assess whether your baby actually seems hungry before you offer a bottle. If they do seem to be hungry? Feed that baby! Always. But if you're not sure? Spending a minute to figure out the true cause of the waking can provide a path for long-term sleep success.

Hunger Signs at Night

Under six months, it is common for babies to wake at night to eat. A hungry baby at night tends to exhibit the following signs: clenched fists, open eyes, rooting reflex if you touch baby's cheek or mouth (baby turns in your direction with an open mouth, looking for a nipple), active sucking on a pacifier or a clean finger, crying upon realizing their sucking isn't leading to milk, and inability to settle when offered nonfeeding soothing methods. If your baby is showing these signs, please feed them! If not, consider that there may be another reason for waking.

Restlessness and Noise

Babies are noisy sleepers. No one warned me about this!

I was completely unprepared for the grunts, sighs, snorts, cries, and whines my babies expressed while sleeping. It freaked me out at first—it didn't seem right! Rest assured that these noises are normal (though if you're unsure, consult with your pediatrician for evaluation). Even wilder? These noises don't tend to wake our babies up. While we jolt awake with a shot of adrenaline hearing a cry, babies often briefly cry out, twitch, and even jerk their arms and legs *in their sleep*. If given a moment to observe before intervening, parents may find that their baby settles and does not continue to cry. If the baby is briefly fussy but not actually awake, picking them up to soothe may create the problem you're attempting to solve—an unhappy, awake baby.

Reasons for Waking

While babies do wake from hunger, there are plenty of other reasons why a baby may wake at night and cry. These can include:

- Wet or dirty (uncomfortable, irritating) diaper

- Temperature that's too hot or cold

- Itchy skin

- Inability to self-soothe

- Inability to put self back to sleep

- Lost pacifier

- Confusion when waking in a different location
  (a crib, for example) from where they fell asleep
  (like your arms)

- Habit

While feeding your baby can feel like the quickest way to get them back to sleep (and it often is, whether or not your baby is hungry—sucking is soothing!), waiting to feed until you assess these other variables can benefit you in the long run.

The Night Feed/Day Snack Cycle

If feeding a baby at night helps *everyone* get back to sleep more quickly, why wouldn't a parent do that? Of course, they could, and many do. However, feeding often at night (particularly when the baby isn't hungry) can thrust the family into a pattern I call the *night feed/day snack cycle*. This occurs when a baby fills up on volume and calories at night, which leads them to take insufficient volume during waking hours, which leads them to seek more calories the next night, and so on. It is thought that this reverse patterning occurs only in breastfed babies, but in my experience, I've seen it with bottle-fed babies, too.

It's relatively easy for a baby to take a full feeding overnight— they're sleepy, there are few distractions, and sucking is soothing. If a parent isn't careful, it can be easy to slide into a pattern where most of your baby's calories are consumed at night, leading them to take smaller "snack" volumes throughout the day. This can continue in a cycle of eating at night until effort is taken to intentionally disrupt it. What I've found is that this disruption process tends to be more painful and takes longer than being careful to avoid the cycle altogether.

I recommend playing the long game, which means stopping to assess whether your baby is actually awake when they cry at night, and then whether there may be another reason for the waking, before you feed. Yes, it may take a few minutes longer than popping a bottle in their mouth, but you will keep yourself out of a habit cycle you likely don't want to be in.

Unsure what to do if your baby wakes at night but isn't hungry? Check out the Quick Tip below for strategies to soothe a waking baby without feeding.

Quick Tip:
Strategies to Try Before Nighttime Feeding

Your baby wakes up crying in the middle of the night, and after you've assessed, you don't think they're hungry. How else do you get them settled and back to sleep? I suggest the following strategies, in order from least intervention to most:

1. **Ensure the room is dark:** Research has shown that babies sleeping in non-dark environments

may get less consolidated sleep and less night-time sleep overall—about half an hour less (and when you're a sleep-deprived parent, every moment counts!). Using room-darkening or light-blocking curtains or blinds is a well-documented strategy to support better sleep for baby.

2. **Wait:** Before you intervene, give your baby a moment or two and see if they settle down without your help. This strategy, referred to in France as *le pause*, means to pause and observe for two to five minutes before taking action. Your baby may put themselves back to sleep during this window without requiring your assistance.

3. **Shush and pat:** If your baby doesn't settle during the pause, try approaching the crib and patting their tummy or backside—note that infants should *always* be placed on their back to sleep and should remain that way until they can independently roll themselves. This patting can provide reassurance (it lets them know someone is attending to them) as well as comfort. You can also check for a stinky diaper at this stage! If they've had a bowel movement, go ahead and change them now. If not, I recom-

mend also shushing while you pat, as this extra white noise (specifically in the whooshing sound familiar to them from the womb) can soothe.

4. **Suck:** Next, introduce a pacifier if your baby will take one. Note that pacifiers are *not* proven to be linked to "nipple confusion" but *are* a protective factor that reduces the likelihood of SIDS. The act of sucking can help calm an agitated baby, so offering a paci while your baby is still in the crib may reduce the likelihood that you'll need to take them out.

5. **Rock:** If it's clear your baby needs to be held, pick them up from the crib and rock them— either by swaying them in your arms or by sitting in a glider or rocking chair. The warmth of your body, your smell, and the motion back and forth may help ease a baby back to sleep without needing to feed.

6. **Change:** If you've tried everything else and your baby still isn't settling down, consider changing their diaper. While this may wake them up further, it also eliminates a potential cause of discomfort that could have led to the night waking in the first place.

Hooray! You've gone through these steps, and now your baby seems content and ready to sleep again. Now for the fun part: Follow the steps in reverse before you put them back in bed. For example, if you changed your baby's diaper (step six), rock them a bit to get them drowsy again (step five), offer a pacifier (step four), stick them in the crib, give them a few pats and shushes (step three), and then wait a few minutes to ensure they're settled (step two). Whatever strategy you landed on—one through six—walk backward from that strategy until you get to "wait," and then leave and enjoy the rest of your night.

While doing "all this" may feel like more work than feeding your baby back to sleep, doing so can help establish quality sleep habits you won't have to break later. And that's called playing the long game!

17

You're Not Crazy: There Is More Spit-Up

I can't tell you the number of messages I get on Instagram and in my email inbox that say something like the following:

My baby has been on the same formula for weeks [or months], and all of a sudden they're spitting up like crazy! Are they now reacting to the formula? Can an allergy develop so late like this? What formula should I try instead?

When I get this message, my first response is always to ask for their baby's age. Almost every time, the parent will tell me their baby is between three (often four) and six months of age. Why is this noteworthy? Because reflux peaks, developmentally, during this time! Most parents, however, aren't aware of this fact. Instead, they go on a wild-goose chase trying different formulas, supplements, and bottles—none of which help because the increase in spit-up is expected and developmentally normal, not caused by something they are doing or a product they are using.

What Is GER?

Gastroesophageal reflux—known as GER, spit-up, or simply reflux—occurs when the contents of the stomach (liquids, foods, and/or stomach acid) come back up into the esophagus and sometimes out of the mouth. In infants, reflux is characterized by an easy flow of liquid—not persistent, and not the forceful vomiting we experience as adults, which is caused by intense muscle contractions in the abdomen. Infant reflux tends to be dribbly versus forceful or projectile and typically does not cause a baby distress or any other symptoms or complications. We often call babies with reflux "happy spitters" because they spit up all day and don't seem to care one bit!

Parents sometimes get concerned about lost calories when an infant has reflux, but the actual spit-up volume is often lower than it appears. Even an ounce of formula or breast milk coming back up will soak a onesie from top to bottom, making it seem like a massive amount of liquid, when in reality, it's typically not as much as it seems. If your baby is still gaining weight appropriately even with increased reflux, they're likely not spitting up a ton of calories—even if it may look like it!

Why Reflux Increases During This Window

While gas tends to peak earlier in infancy and reduce by the three-month mark, reflux tends to get worse. This can be confusing for new parents who thought their baby's digestive system was finally maturing! There are a few reasons why we tend to see more spit-up between three and six months of age:

1. **Higher-volume feedings.** Infants often go through a growth spurt at three months and again at six months. During these times, the volume of breast milk or formula that your baby is taking in will likely increase. While this increase in the number of feedings or ounces daily helps support their rapid growth, it also means there's more liquid volume sitting in the baby's belly.

2. **Increased movement.** By this time, your baby is becoming much more interested in the world around them. They have sharper visual acuity, more control over their limbs, and may be eager to explore! Additionally, some babies will start to roll, scoot, or even crawl during this window, and these activities increase both time and pressure on the belly. Increased movement, especially movement where your baby isn't in an upright position, combined with the larger volume of liquid intake, is a recipe for more spit-up.

3. **Esophageal sphincter weakness.** That's right! The band of muscle at the bottom of the esophagus (the lower esophageal sphincter) is *still* developing during this age range. This may mean it isn't as effective at preventing reflux. Until it gains more strength, the likelihood of reflux remains higher.

4. **Lack of solids.** The American Academy of Pediatrics recommends parents start solid foods nearer to the six-month mark than the four-month mark. Introduction of solids, such as infant cereal, may be recommended by your child's pediatrician if your child has reflux. Talk to your pediatrician about when to start solids and whether introducing them can be a method for managing symptoms of reflux.

When GER Is Actually GERD

For many babies, reflux is nothing more than a transient annoyance—and mostly for mom and/or dad. For some, however, reflux is severe enough to be classified as GERD, or gastroesophageal reflux disease. Symptoms of GERD can include recurrent regurgitation with or without vomiting, slow or inadequate weight gain, bottle refusal or refusal to nurse, wheezing, and general discomfort or agitation. If your baby is experiencing these symptoms along with frequent, hard-to-control spit-up—or if they are having any other symptoms you find concerning—talk to your pediatrician about whether it may be GERD versus "happy spitting" versus any other disorders. In this case, different strategies may be used to treat it.

Speaking of strategies, check the Quick Tip below for a list of methods to try if you want to attempt to reduce how often your baby spits up. I can't promise a miracle, but they are worth a try—promise.

Quick Tip:
Tools for Managing Reflux

As discussed above, gastrointestinal reflux can be developmentally normal and doesn't necessarily indicate a problem, even if it occurs frequently. What is a problem, however, is the sheer amount of laundry that comes with a spitty baby! Avoiding this alone is worth trying to solve the reflux puzzle. Along with discussing with your pediatrician, here are my top tips for managing reflux if you have a spitty baby:

Wait It Out: For better and for worse, babies change quickly. Most reflux resolves on its own as a baby gets older and their digestive system (including the lower esophageal sphincter) matures. If the laundry doesn't bother you, and your baby is gaining weight appropriately and experiencing no other problems, you can choose to wait and assume their reflux will resolve over time.

Use Paced Feeding Techniques: If you remember from chapter 8, granting your baby more control of their milk intake by feeding them in an upright position may make a difference. When feeding, make sure your baby is upright and the bottle is relatively level so that they can control the flow of milk and better coordinate their sucking, breathing, and swallowing, as this is thought to be helpful.

Avoid Overfeeding: I'm sure this is attributable to someone other than my dad, but in our family, he's basically got the phrase trademarked—*If you overfeed them, they overflow.* It makes sense, right? Too much volume in the belly has a tendency to come back up. We experience this as adults, too! I always suggest being conservative in how much you feed your baby, because you can always offer more if they still show hunger signs when they've had what you offered (see the Quick Tip for the "top-up bottle" trick). It's better to start small and add volume as needed, because once they've consumed too much milk, there's no way to take it back.

Get Out a Good Burp: Some babies are better burpers than others! If you have a baby with reflux, working to help them burp effectively is crucial. Not only does this reduce the discomfort of trapped gas in the tummy, letting that air escape early after a feeding can help limit reflux later. While many people default to burping their baby by patting their baby's back while they're over the shoulder, this isn't the only way to get them to burp. Sitting your baby upright (on your thigh, for example) while supporting their chin with one hand and pushing up on their back with the other (they should get "taller" as their spine lengthens with the gentle push upward) can also result in a burp. Doing bicycle legs and baby massages can also help your baby release air that may otherwise lead to reflux, though I don't suggest doing this shortly after a feeding, because it tends to require a reclined position.

Keep 'Em Upright: This may be the most frequently discussed of reflux strategies, but it's repeated often because it works! Keeping a baby upright after feeding (for up to sixty minutes) gives the digestive system time to process their meal. The time it takes for liquids to leave the stomach—called *gastric emptying*—varies depending on the age of the child and how much they're fed at a given time. Infants between the ages of three to six months demonstrate an average of about 42 percent gastric emptying one hour after a meal and an average of about 91 percent gastric emptying three hours after a meal. While it takes time to digest, know that nearly half of their meal may pass through their stomach within the first hour! Giving your baby time for their breast milk or formula to move out of the stomach means that when you eventually lay them down to play or eat, there's less volume in the belly that can splash back up.

Ensure Correct Nipple Flow: Reflux's favorite friend is extra air. Ensuring you have the correct nipple flow for your baby's bottle—not too slow and not too fast—can reduce unnecessary air intake during feeding. Unsure if your baby's nipple flow rate is right? Check chapter 11 for guidance. While we're discussing swallowed air, it's also worth mentioning that extra pacifier time may be a culprit. Try less pacifier time, if you can.

Tried these strategies above with no luck? You can also explore the following under the guidance of your child's pediatrician or care team:

Consider OTC Remedies: Step into Walgreens or CVS and you will see a whole shelf of infant supplements that claim to tackle gas, fussiness, and reflux.

Supplements are not regulated as stringently as infant formulas, and therefore, all include a disclaimer that says something like, "These statements have not been evaluated by the Food and Drug Administration. This product is not intended to diagnose, treat, cure, or prevent any disease." Common supplements that parents might try for gas or reflux include probiotics (some research exists to support their benefit), gas drops that contain simethicone (although there isn't adequate evidence to support its use), and gripe water containing a blend of "soothing" herbs like ginger and fennel (again, there isn't adequate evidence to support its use). Please discuss these options with your pediatrician before use, as some supplements may not be appropriate for some babies.

Try a Hypoallergenic Formula: For a subset of babies with cow milk protein allergy (CMPA), reflux is the only clear indicator. If your little one has reflux that cannot be managed with the usual strategies, trying a hypoallergenic (extensively hydrolyzed) formula may help.

Assess for Oral Restrictions or Other Oral Motor Issues: The most underutilized resource in infant feeding, in my opinion, is a well-trained speech-language pathologist (SLP) who specializes in babies. Many parents overlook this option, as the name *speech-language pathologist* doesn't seem to apply to infants who can't talk yet! The key here is that SLPs are trained to diagnose and correct dysfunction in the muscles in the mouth. Sometimes this looks like training an older child to put their tongue in the correct position when making an S sound, but this skill set is also applicable for evaluating whether a baby's mouth and tongue are operating the way they should to eat effectively and efficiently. If you can't figure out your baby's reflux, setting up a consultation with a pediatric SLP can be a great place to start.

Use a Thickening Agent: In generations past, the recommendation was to thicken a baby's milk by adding infant cereal or oatmeal to their bottle—both to help reduce reflux and to help them sleep. While this practice is no longer recommended for sleep, the use of thickeners is still recommended for a subset of babies who experience gastroesophageal reflux. Oatmeal is thought to be a safe source for thickening, as is Gelmix, a carob bean–based thickener approved for use in infants after forty-two weeks gestational age. Talk to your child's pediatrician about thickeners, especially about how to arrive at the just-right consistency to support reflux management, while being mindful of developmental readiness (you want your baby to be able to handle the thickening) and the avoidance of overfeeding (as thickeners will provide added carbohydrates and calories).

Try Reflux Medication: If all else fails, you may have luck with medication, although I recommend this strategy last, as it doesn't consider or address the root cause of the reflux—and because you may first find benefit with non-pharmacologic options. Medications called *histamine type-2 receptor antagonists* (like famotidine and ranitidine) and *proton pump inhibitors* (like lansoprazole and omeprazole) work by reducing or neutralizing stomach acid to treat symptoms. But even experts recommend that they be used only in certain situations, so be sure to discuss their use with your child's pediatrician.

Remember, reflux is common and tends to improve with age. While the strategies shared here may provide some relief, rest assured that there will come a day in the future when your baby is no longer a baby and you no longer have to deal with infant spit-up. In that moment, you might even miss it (or you won't, let's be real).

Mom Note

For the Mom Who Wanted to Breastfeed, but Couldn't

Allow me to be vulnerable and share some of the ways my body isn't perfect:

- My eyes don't see very well.

- My joints are floppy because my connective tissue is defective (a genetic condition).

- My skin punctures easily and then heals imperfectly, leaving scars.

- My pancreas is more likely than not to crap out on me after two rounds of gestational diabetes.

- My brain needs help balancing various neurotransmitters, which leaves me prone to anxiety and depression.

The reality is that my body, like most, doesn't always work perfectly, or as it "should."

Can we agree that none of what I've said so far is controversial? It's an accepted part of the human condition that our bodies are fallible. And on the whole—thankfully—we don't tend to ascribe moral value to our bodies working the right way. It simply is what it is, particularly as we age. We expect that our bodies won't function the way we want them to as we get older, and while we feel bad about it, we don't tend to feel that we are *bad people* because of it.

For example, while I grieve the loss of certain freedoms as a result of having poor vision, I don't feel like I've done something *wrong* by having bad eyesight. Having less than twenty-twenty vision doesn't feel like a reflection of my goodness as a person. Sometimes our body parts work like they should; other times they don't. I don't hide the fact that my body is less than perfect in this area, because I'm not embarrassed by it. I wear my glasses and it's fine.

So why, then, do so many of us feel ashamed and embarrassed when we can't breastfeed?

I believe it's because we have ingested the narrative—popular on social media—that our worthiness is tied to how much milk we can produce and for how long.

There's a phrase that often circulates within mom spaces on the internet regarding birth and breastfeeding: *Your body was made to do this.*

It's a nice enough sentiment, but it neglects the fundamental truth that so often, our bodies do not function the way they were "made to." And when we experience this personally, the question we have to reckon with is, "What, and who, do I believe when my body doesn't cooperate like I want, or like I believe it should?"

Social media feeds us plenty of thinly veiled ideas when it comes to breastfeeding and/or producing breast milk, and many are harmful. Sentiments like:

- *If your body doesn't work right, you did something wrong.*

- *If you can't breastfeed, you didn't try hard enough.*

- *If only you truly believed in your body's innate power, you would've been successful.*

- *If you did your homework, you'd know that low supply is very, very rare, so you likely don't actually have a problem, even if your doctor told you otherwise.*

- *You probably could've breastfed if only you X, Y, or Z . . .*

I call bullshit. Sometimes the answer is that bodies don't work super well. No different from any of the myriad other ways our bodies can let us down. And yet we don't believe, or tolerate, these phrases about any other limitation. Could you imagine these phrases above being used in another context? *If you really believed in your ability to produce lactase enzymes, you wouldn't be lactose intolerant. Your body was made to produce them! You aren't trying hard enough!* Ridiculous, right? We wouldn't accept someone saying this to a loved one of ours, and yet, so often we say a version of this to ourselves when it comes to making milk.

Leaning into the example of how we talk or feel about *other* limitations can help us reframe our beliefs and remove the shame some feel about using formula.

Here's what I mean.

When our bodies don't work the way they should, we (the brilliant, resourceful species we are!) create accommodations:

- Glasses or contacts for poor eyesight.

- Artificial limbs for people with amputations.

- Insulin pumps for people with diabetes.

- Ostomy bags for people with severe inflammatory bowel disease.

- Medication for mental health.

The list goes on and on.

The purpose of these accommodations is to *promote functioning*. No one argues about whether these solutions are as good as the "real thing." In many cases, they're not. In other cases, they are. But that's not the point, is it? The point is to promote an as-close-as-possible *functional outcome* for the person who needs it.

And we not only tolerate these interventions, we often celebrate them as wins for the human condition. These are triumphs of science! We express gratitude that we live in such a time that we have options for bodies that don't work optimally; options that allow people to participate as fully as possible with their (our) imperfections.

Political correctness (and basic human decency) dictates

that we not malign people who take advantage of accommodations to help them or their bodies function. No one shouts, "Flesh is best!" to a person with a prosthetic leg. Of course, we all know having two working human legs is ideal. But gosh, what a gift that we have a solution for those without a functioning leg that provides the ability to walk and stand.

No one shouts, "Twenty-twenty is best!" to a person with glasses. Of course, we all know having perfect vision is ideal. But what a gift to have a solution for those with nearsightedness or farsightedness or astigmatism (that's me!) that provides the ability to see.

We can claim this same narrative when it comes to using formula. We can know that breast milk offers ideal nutrition for infants *and* acknowledge that we don't always live in ideal bodies (and this is true of both ourselves and our babies, as sometimes it's *their* anatomy that creates the challenge). We can believe formula is a gift for those who want or need it as a means to provide the ability to nourish babies. Baby formula provides the same function as breast milk: complete nutrition that supports healthy growth and development for infants, even though it's not identical.

Thinking about formula in this light was intensely helpful in my journey of dropping guilt and shame around my "failed" breastfeeding journey. Formula is a tool, like so many others, that helped me function when my body didn't.

Using formula doesn't say anything about me, just like using glasses doesn't say anything about me.

My set of slacker boobs are no more a moral failing than my hypermobile elbows.

Getting diagnosed with postpartum depression isn't worthy of judgment any more than getting diagnosed with a complete placenta previa during pregnancy (which didn't move—shout-out to my C-section mamas).

We can choose to believe that having a body that is sometimes unpredictable or uncooperative is part of the human experience, not a moral failure, and that using the accommodations we have available to us is a win, not a compromise.

We can reject the belief that not breastfeeding, or not producing enough milk, or not producing milk for a certain prescribed time period is somehow the ultimate moral failure.

This doesn't mean we ignore real feelings that may accompany a feeding journey that doesn't go as planned. Feelings of disappointment, grief, frustration, jealousy, and so many others are common. Instead, this means that we treat ourselves—and our bodies—the same way in this area that we do in others, which is with a lot more grace, kindness, and neutrality.

The human body doesn't always cooperate, yes, but we have work-arounds. And thank goodness for that.

6–9 Months

18

Milk Stays King!
Balancing Food and Formula

Starting solids is exciting! Often, parents jump in headfirst and start offering meals, snacks, smoothies, and all sorts of things the minute their baby turns six months old. Before you do that, please remember this:

For the entirety of your baby's first year, milk (formula or breast milk) is the most important source of nutrition, not just the first six months!

Solids—in any format—are complementary during a baby's first year. After the introduction of solid foods when your baby is developmentally ready (which is usually around six months of age), they will gradually transition to consuming more solids and less milk (formula or breast milk). By their first birthday, most babies are ready to consume a healthy eating pattern, which includes age-appropriate foods complemented by milk (such as cow's milk, breast milk, or a milk alternative). Until then, milk stays king, with a recommended daily intake of twenty-four to thirty-two ounces a day until twelve months.

Why Prioritize Milk?

Breast milk and formula offer ideal nutrition for infants from zero to twelve months. Crucially, both liquids are nutrient dense. In the United States, formulas for full-term, healthy infants usually offer around one hundred calories—plus roughly two grams of protein, five grams of fat, and ten to eleven grams of carbohydrates—per five-ounce bottle, although this can vary. This bottle is packed with nutrition!

Consider green beans, on the other hand. A serving of pureed green beans (four ounces) from a leading baby food manufacturer clocks in at forty calories, zero grams of fat, and one gram of protein. Alternatively, a cup of cooked green beans is only thirty calories. If you substitute a bottle feeding for a serving of green beans, your baby will receive a much lower volume of macronutrients than they would from their breast milk or formula. This is why we want solids to complement milk feedings at this stage—not replace them.

Additionally, it can be hard to measure how much of a serving of solids your baby actually eats. Solids, especially when you allow your baby to self-serve, are notorious for ending up in their hair, smeared on the tray of their high chair, and all over the floor. Because the first year is a crucial developmental period, we want to ensure our babies are getting all the calories, fat, protein, carbs, and micronutrients they need to grow well!

If Formula Provides Adequate Nutrition, Why Introduce Solids at All?

This is not to say that solids aren't important during your baby's first year. They are! Solids are important for providing nutrients to your baby, along with giving them exposure to different flavors, textures, and types of foods. Offering your baby solids helps them develop:

- Fine motor skills (moving from the palmer grasp to the pincer grasp as they learn to pick up smaller bites of food or grasp a spoon)

- Hand-eye coordination

- Oral motor skills and tongue coordination

- Muscle strength in the mouth and jaw

- Familiarity and comfort with different food groups

- Social skills as they participate in mealtimes with their caregivers

Solids serve as an important companion to the nutrition that is found within formula (or breast milk), and they offer

an important developmental function during a baby's first
year of life, too.

Keeping Milk in Charge

To maintain breast milk or formula as the primary source of
nutrition for your baby while introducing solid foods, consider a few guidelines.

First, you don't have to jump immediately to offering three
meals and two snacks a day with your six-month-old baby! I
recommend one meal of solids per day at six and seven months,
two meals of solids per day at eight, nine, and ten months, and
three meals of solids per day at eleven and twelve months, since
this helps with a gradual transition. I rarely introduced snacks
during my babies' first year, although you may find that introducing one or two per day works well for your baby! Within
a few months of starting solids, your baby should be eating a
variety of developmentally appropriate foods at a variety of
meal and/or snack times. This could include formula and/
or breast milk, vegetables, fruits, proteins like eggs and fish,
grains like oatmeal, and fats like avocados and (appropriately
thinned out) nut butters.

Second, consider offering a milk feeding before or alongside each meal of solids, and remember to engage in responsive
feeding. That means listening to your baby's hunger and fullness cues—allowing them to eat when they're hungry and stop
when they show signs of satiety. Allow your baby to choose
how much and whether to eat the foods that you offer. And
if at first they throw all their food on the floor or spit out
their puree, know that it can take repeated exposure to solids

before the new flavors and textures become acceptable. Keep listening and keep trying!

Third, if you notice your baby is experiencing slow weight gain as a result of introducing solids, talk to your pediatrician about introducing nutrient-rich foods with higher calories, such as those with a greater amount of healthy fats. If you notice a decrease in milk volume but your baby is still growing well, meeting milestones, and maintaining (roughly) their growth curve, you may be advised that the lower milk intake is fine for their age.

Bottom Line

We know solids are exciting for babies and parents alike! They are colorful, flavorful, and novel compared to the same milk day after day, and they represent an important introduction to family mealtimes. While formula or breast milk will play a leading role until a child turns one, starting solids during the first year sets a strong foundation for successful eating after the first birthday.

Quick Tip:

How to Use Formula in Food

Did you know any recipe that includes milk can be made with formula instead? I've been known to use baby formula in place of cow's milk in my kids' Kraft mac and cheese, and they're none the wiser! (Note: This is not a formal recommendation, and I do not want to receive social media messages if your kids think it's nasty. Try it at your own risk!) Parents may choose to add formula into other foods for a variety of reasons, including:

1. Convenience—formula is shelf-stable, and many parents already have it on hand.

2. Nutrition—formula is fortified with a larger variety of nutrients compared to cow's milk.

3. Tolerance—for infants with cow milk protein allergy, a hypoallergenic formula that's well tolerated can be used as a substitute for milk (though I cannot guarantee it will make the recipe taste good).

4. Texture—if a certain puree is too thick for your baby (for example, peanut butter), formula can be used to thin it to a desired consistency.

If you want to use formula in or with other foods, keep in mind our formula food safety rules (see chapter 7). This means not leaving food made with formula out for more than two hours at room temperature and not consuming it after twenty-four hours if stored in the fridge. I should point out that, when using formula in this way, it could be harder to measure how much was actually consumed—though precise measuring and monitoring at this age may not be as important as it was in the earlier months, provided your baby is growing appropriately. Once solids are introduced, you may find that your baby drinks more formula one day and less another. This can be okay.

Another consideration is that high temperatures (like used for baking) can degrade some of the nutrients in the formula, changing the nutrition per serving from what is stated on the formula container's label. You'll also want to be sure that your baby has reached the appropriate developmental milestones before introducing foods (including foods made with formula).

Here are a few of my favorite ways to use formula in foods!

Cereals: Rice cereal and/or baby oatmeal can be good options for infants, as they are fortified with iron—and infants need plenty of iron during the second half of their first year! Follow instructions on the back of the infant cereal package to mix, using prepared formula in place of water. Note that the AAP recommends oatmeal over rice cereal due to concerns about repeated exposure to arsenic found in rice during the developmental period of infancy.

Smoothies: Add prepared formula along with fruits and veggies into a blender and whip up a glass of nutrition! You can even add avocado for extra healthy fats. Smoothies are a fun way to sneak in extra nutrients from non-preferred foods.

Smoothie pops: Have extra smoothie left over in the blender? Freeze it in an ice pop tray! These smoothie pops can be perfect for hot summer days or cranky teething babies (try plopping them in the bathtub with the pop to reduce mess—my kids still request a "Popsicle bath" from time to time). Note that formula, on its own, should not be frozen, and formula frozen in a smoothie may not retain the same nutrients at the same volumes it has unfrozen. Use ice pops within four months of freezing.

French toast: Grab a slice of wheat bread, an egg, prepared formula, a dash of cinnamon, and a dash of (alcohol-free) vanilla extract. Whisk the egg, add a bit of formula to thin it, add the cinnamon and vanilla for flavor, and soak the bread in the mixture. Cook the slice in a skillet until it's brown on both sides! For infants, there's no need to serve with syrup. Instead, you've got fiber, protein, and a bunch of micronutrients without the excess sugar.

Nut butters: Peanut butter and almond butter, on their own, are too thick for infants and are considered a choking hazard. We know, however, that early and frequent exposure to allergens like peanuts and tree nuts is important to reduce the risk of food allergies! One of my favorite methods for introduction? Use formula to thin the nut butter into a liquid consistency and then drizzle on top of yogurt. If you leave it a bit thicker, you can spread it on top of crackers or teething wafers as well.

While these are some of my top ideas, you can get creative here! I know parents who have baked formula into their baby's first birthday cakes, used it to soften corn flakes that their baby can then pick up to eat, and added it to pasta sauces. If you have it on hand and want to use it in place of milk, go for it!

Mom Note

Every Choice You Make Is Wrong (History Proves It)

I don't have many favorite photos of myself as an infant. This is not my parents' fault! They have plenty of pictures tucked behind sticky, yellowing plastic in albums with tufted fabric covers. As an identical twin, my issue is how often I'm unsure if a photo I'm looking at is actually of *me*. If you're not a twin, let me tell you—it's a disorienting experience not being able to accurately identify yourself in a photo. I don't recommend it. But back to the point. I tell you this because one of my favorite pictures from infancy has a baby—on the back, it says ten months old—in a car seat with no chest clip, facing forward, in the *front* seat of a car. For the sake of this essay, let's decide that the baby in the front seat is me.

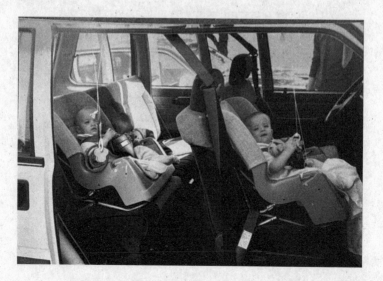

When I first stumbled upon this picture several years ago, I was horrified. Can you imagine? There are *so* many safety issues documented in the image! A parent could probably be arrested for securing a baby like that today. We now know that kids should ride in rear-facing car seats for as long as possible (until they reach the top height or weight limit allowed by the manufacturer) and that the back seat of the car is best until a child is at least twelve years of age (or as otherwise required by state law). Looking back at the photo of me as a baby in the front seat, the whole thing feels reckless—negligent, even. How could they think that was okay?

The answer is that parents do the best they can with the knowledge they have at the time . . . but knowledge changes over time.

My parents, in the mid-1980s, were following all the guidelines that existed for car and car seat safety. They felt as confident in their choices then as I feel now when I buckle my kids in—maybe more so, as they didn't have social media to make them second-guess every parenting decision they ever made. They made the best choices available to them at the time. Thirty-some years later, though, we can look back and say, with clarity, that these particular choices are no longer best.

This pattern repeats itself over and over again if you look at how recommendations from health agencies have changed over time. Adding rice cereal to bottles to help babies sleep? This was common practice in the '80s and '90s and is expressly discouraged now. Introducing solids as early as six weeks? Now the recommendation is around six months. Using a drop-side crib? They can no longer be sold due to safety concerns. As time goes on, recommendations change based on new information. What was once "best" quickly becomes "not best," and sometimes even "downright dangerous" as our collective knowledge grows.

This means, almost certainly, that whatever choice you're agonizing over right now in your parenting journey will be looked back on unfavorably by future generations—even if you make the "right choice" today.

While some parents may argue that this knowledge makes our current efforts meaningless (*What's the point if it's all going to be wrong someday?*), I think it provides freedom. Knowing the choices we make today are "doing the best we can with the information we have" decisions and not "the be-all and end-all of raising a baby into a successful, healthy, and happy adult" takes the pressure off.

If we have the privilege of living for several more decades, we will undoubtedly watch as the choices we made for our babies—with excruciating care, hours of research, and sometimes plenty of tears—fall out of favor with disgust. This is simply the nature of progress and how recommendations evolve over time. It would be hubris to assume that our generation has somehow reached the pinnacle of correctness while all others prior fell short.

Remember—they thought they were correct, too.

Given this, my approach for handling fraught parenting decisions has changed. Previously, my approach was white-knuckling everything because of the belief that I had one chance to get this right or else my baby wouldn't reach their full potential and it would be entirely my fault. Now, my approach is:

None of these options is likely going to be "right" in the future, so which one feels best for me today *based on what I know and what's important to me?*

This framework can apply to any of the choices that bog parents down in the first year of their baby's life, as well as those after, including:

- Breastfeeding or formula feeding

- Purees or baby-led weaning

- Sleep training or no sleep training

- Staying home full-time or working outside the home

- Day care or a nanny

- Private school or public school

- Screen time or no screen time

The goal can't be to "make no wrong choices." This is unattainable and maddening. The reality is many—if not all—of the choices we make today will turn out to be wrong decades from now. Let this be a comfort to you! Doing the best we can with the information we have is the only way forward in parenting—then, now, and always.

19

There Are a Million Right Ways to Start Solids

Spend any amount of time on "momstagram"—the collo-
quial name for mom-related content on Instagram—and
you will find more advice, opinions, and instructions about
introducing solid foods to your baby than you could ever attempt to consume (pun intended, I think). There are a few
trains of thought when it comes to starting solids, and they
tend to exist in opposition to one another. Each strategy pur-
ports to offer what parents want—safety and/or less risk of
choking, reduced likelihood of pickiness in toddlerhood, appropriate oral motor development, and exposure to a variety
of macronutrients and vitamins and minerals. As a result, the

risk of making the "wrong" choice feels high. No one wants to wonder, down the line, if their toddler's refusal to eat vegetables when they are two and a half is the result of doing solids wrong in infancy!

So what's a parent to do? As with everything else, the only thing you *can* do is evaluate your options, think through your own personal goals and preferences, and remind yourself that your child's outcomes in this area (like so many others!) will occur not only because of your efforts but also in spite of them. There is no single "right way" to introduce solids, and in fact, there may be a million "right ways" based on the unique needs of your family. Even better, there are only a few wrong ways, and they are easy to avoid. Let's go through them!

Frameworks for Solid Introduction

Purees: For many years, introducing soft, pureed food was the go-to method for starting solids in infancy. Pediatricians used to advise starting with rice cereal, as this is a smooth, mild option that also provides iron. After that, parents were advised to move to pureed vegetables (because of the belief that fruit may condition the palate to prefer sweet foods), then fruits, then pureed meats and combinations of all three. If you visit the baby food aisle of any major grocery store today, you will find all these options and more, each featuring different ingredients and textures.

While pureed foods are not always the default method of introducing solids these days, many parents still prefer to start with them. They can offer ease and potentially cleaner meal-times. Packaged purees can be a good option for convenience (I used them with both of our kids), while some parents may prefer to make their own. Purees also don't have to be fancy! Mashing up single-ingredient foods, like avocado or steamed carrots that you may already have on hand, also counts.

If you decide to offer purees, you can get creative with the presentation. Purees can be spread on crackers or whole wheat toast, drizzled over or mixed with other foods, and pre-placed on a training spoon to allow your baby to practice feeding him- or herself. Gone are the days when purees meant solely airplane-spooning the mush into your baby's waiting mouth!

Single-ingredient introduction: Current guidance from the AAP and CDC recommends introducing new single-ingredient foods to your baby one at a time and waiting three to five days to watch for reactions before introducing the next food. But allergy experts suggest that this practice may not be necessary, as it may prolong exposure of other new foods. We know that early allergen introduction and consistent exposure is important! Parents should watch for signs of a reaction when top allergens—like peanuts, tree nuts, cow's milk products, eggs, fish, shellfish, wheat, soy, and sesame—are served.

Baby-led weaning: In the last five to ten years, we've seen a major social push toward a method of solids introduction called *baby-led weaning*. The name is a bit of a misnomer, as the goal, when starting solids at around six months of age, is not to wean entirely from breast milk or formula in exchange for food but rather to continue to breast or formula feed while offering solids! The more important piece here is the concept of *baby-led*. Baby-led weaning, in practice, often means offering table foods, cut or modified to be baby-safe in size and shape, that your little one can feed to themselves. This approach puts the baby in control of whether to eat what's offered and, if so, how much—summarized as, "Parent provides, baby decides." Often, this is referred to as *division of responsibility* in feeding, and some research suggests that it reduces the parent's pressure on their child to eat throughout toddlerhood.

If you decide to follow the baby-led weaning approach for starting solids, be sure to educate yourself on safe preparation of foods by baby age. For example, steak is best served to babies at six months in a long strip (or on a bone) that they can gnaw on. By nine months, when babies have more teeth and stronger jaw muscles, steak should be served shredded to reduce choking risk. My favorite resource to learn about safe food preparation and presentation for infants is the organization Solid Starts, which has an app, a social media presence, and a book that can be easily referenced.

100 foods before 1: Some parents set a goal for how many unique foods they want to offer their baby before the first birthday. The "100 foods before 1" approach is thought to help reduce picky eating by offering your baby exposure to a wide variety of foods. Doing this also guarantees that your baby has access to the wide variety of vitamins and minerals contained in those different foods. For some, this framework provides a guide that can ease parental stress, as it lays out what to do and which foods to offer. For others, this could increase worry, as it may be difficult for some to source and prepare so many different foods in a short time frame, and parents don't want to feel like they've "failed" if they don't reach one hundred foods.

My Recommendation?
The "Best of Everything" Approach

Circling back to the top, there isn't one singular correct way to do solids with your baby. Instead, I recommend (as I do with basically everything) to create a system that works for you, your goals, and the needs of your family. This may look like baby-led weaning at dinner and pureed pouches on the go. It can mean store-bought baby food with a side of soft vegetables from your lunch. You can set a goal of fifty foods instead of one hundred by the first birthday, or you can decide not to track foods at all (I didn't)! If allergies are a special source of worry, ask your child's pediatrician if your baby would be considered at higher risk and form a plan from there. I had a friend who introduced peanut butter in her car in the children's hospital parking lot just in case. (I'm not saying this is advisable or necessary, but rather it's an example that you can do whatever you want!)

You can also modify your approach as your baby ages, or with future children if you have them. You can change what you're doing if you try one method and it doesn't work for you. The ultimate goal is that your baby is exposed to a variety of tastes and textures and has the opportunity to practice picking up food, chewing it, and manipulating it in their mouth. How you get there is up to you! As always, if you have questions or concerns about starting solids, talking with your pediatrician is the best place to start.

Solids No-Nos

Hopefully, you are now convinced there isn't a single right way to introduce solids. I'm so glad! There are, however, a few things to avoid as you begin adding table food to your baby's diet.

Honey: The AAP recommends avoiding honey under the age of one due to risk of botulism, a rare but serious type of food poisoning—especially for infants (as they have less developed immune systems). Honey can contain *Clostridium botulinum* bacteria, and when consumed, these bacteria spores produce toxins. It's important to know that this bacteria can be found in both pasteurized and raw honey, so best practice is to avoid honey altogether during your child's infancy.

Processed foods with added sugar and/or high in salt: It's recommended to give infants whole, minimally processed foods, as some packaged and processed foods can contain added sugars or alternative sweeteners and high levels of sodium. Additionally, sugar-sweetened beverages and fruit juices are not recommended under age one—stick to water and formula or breast milk.

High-mercury fish: While fish can be a great source of protein and DHA (an omega-3 fatty acid) for infants, it's recommended to avoid fish that contain higher levels of mercury, such as swordfish, marlin, tilefish, and king mackerel. Salmon, shrimp, flounder, and haddock are good choices that contain less mercury! Pay attention to serving size and suggested serving frequency by age as well.

Choking hazards: While most foods can be prepared and

served safely for infants, there are a few popular foods that you should pay particular attention too—or avoid altogether—until your baby is older. These include popcorn, uncut grapes and cherry tomatoes (instead, slice into quarters longways), whole or chopped nuts, hot dogs (slice into strips instead of leaving whole or cutting into rounds or coins), certain candies, and un-thinned nut butters. Children, especially those under the age of four, are still learning how to chew and swallow. By preparing foods safely—for example, by cutting some foods into appropriately sized pieces and by cooking hard foods (like carrots) until they are soft—you can help reduce the risk of their small airways becoming blocked. Continue to follow recommendations about safe preparation (or safe introduction age) for foods that are commonly known to be choking hazards, and be sure to supervise your baby as they learn to master their new chewing skills.

You Can Do It!

Introducing solids can come with some apprehension for new parents. Remember that learning to eat table food is truly that—a learning process. You don't need to jump in and go wild the first day, or even the first few months, of your baby's second half of infancy. With continued exposure, opportunity, and practice, both you and your baby are likely to become more comfortable with solids, which will increase enjoyment of mealtimes for everybody.

Quick Tip:
I'll Have What You're Having

Baby food doesn't have to be complicated! One of the best tips for starting your baby on solids is to offer them—in an age-appropriate size and shape—whatever you're eating for your meal. The method that worked best for our family is something I call *meal deconstruction*. Here are a few examples:

- If I'm eating cereal for breakfast, I can give my baby some cereal pieces that have been softened in almond milk to an appropriate texture.

- If I'm eating eggs, I can serve some scrambled to my baby (add cheese for dairy exposure, if desired!).

- If I'm eating beef stew, I can serve my baby shreds of beef, plus cooked carrots and potatoes (smashed or cut).

- If I'm eating a salad, I can give my baby cheese shreds, plus tomatoes and cucumbers (cut appropriately) from the top before I mix in the dressing.

- If I'm eating a hamburger, I can tear off pieces of ground beef and pieces of bun, and let my baby have a french fry or two.

- If I'm making spaghetti, I can give my baby some noodles and smash up a meatball into smaller chunks.

You don't need to make special food for your baby! It is likely that your baby can eat whatever the rest of the family is eating—the key is to make sure it's served in a way that reduces choking risk.

But What If *My* Diet Is Terrible?

This was a question I wrestled with, as I have been known (even as I approach forty) to eat a bag of Doritos and a Reese's cup as the occasional breakfast. Obviously, I'm not going to serve that to my baby for his first meal of the day! I found that having a baby to share my food with increased how often I was cooking and eating well-rounded meals, as I wanted my baby to eat better than I typically did. This was a win for me! I also chose to supplement my baby's meals with store-bought baby food (typically veggie-based) so my baby got daily servings of vegetables even if I didn't (I'm really telling on myself here).

I'd also encourage you to think about your baby's diet on a weekly basis versus daily. It's okay if some days aren't "great" in terms of getting in all the servings of each food group. Look at the larger picture and assess whether your baby's diet looks pretty good at the weekly level—it very well might. Lastly, give yourself grace. It's okay to hide in the pantry and eat chocolate or drive through Taco Bell occasionally for yourself and then give your baby more well-rounded leftovers at home. We want to be mindful—not perfect—when it comes to our eating and our baby's.

Mom Note
"Fed Is Best" Applies to Table Food, Too!

The original name for this essay was "French Fries Are a Vegetable!" but it got shot down during edits. The fact remains, however, that potatoes *are* a vegetable, and slicing and frying them doesn't negate this truth. Honestly, if you're in the South, mac and cheese is considered a vegetable at most "meat and three" restaurants, so the french fry example doesn't feel like a stretch! I digress. The point is this: The goal is a *fed* baby, not a *perfectly fed* baby, and sometimes a fed baby may mean offering french fries (or whatever other "less healthy" food they will eat).

The Ideal

Infancy (and later, toddlerhood) is a crucial developmental period, and access to quality foods that offer a variety of nutrients is important. The AAP suggests offering foods like avocado, dairy (yogurt and cottage cheese), eggs, fish, whole grains, and nut butters (appropriately thinned to reduce choking risk). Infants are also recommended to consume fruits and vegetables daily, and for good reason—increased consumption of fruits and vegetables in late infancy is associated with increased likelihood of eating fruits and vegetables at age six! The habits we start when our babies are infants can set the stage for continued good eating habits later in life.

We also know, however, that babies don't always subscribe to expert recommendations like we want them to. And in this case, please remember:

"Fed is best," as a statement and sentiment, applies to table food, too.

There's no rule that says at nine or twelve months we have to throw out our belief that "fed is best." It would be a pity to work hard during the first year of our baby's life to feel unashamed of formula feeding . . . only to turn around and feel bad about offering convenience food occasionally or not consistently serving five vegetables a day. I believe that every parent who's feeding a baby—and then later, a toddler—does their best with the resources they have (time, money, access to stores, etc.). Often, our resources constrain us and make it difficult to meet the pie-in-the-sky vision of grinding our own flour to make our own crackers. This is okay! *Fed is best.*

The Reality: Your Kid Needs to Eat

My mom and I were chatting recently about how picky my twin sister and I were in our early years (we've gotten less so over time, thankfully). She recalled a conversation she had with my grandmother where she huffed, "I don't know what to do! The only things these girls will eat are white carbs!" And my grandma, in her infinite wisdom after raising three kids of her own, replied, "Then feed them white carbs. It won't be forever." She was right. Sometimes, the answer is to feed your kid what they will eat, often by including a preferred food on their plate and surrounding it with other foods for exposure. They may only eat the thing they like, but that's okay. They've eaten, and you've created an opportunity for them to explore beyond that. It takes an estimated ten to fifteen exposures of a new food before a baby might try it!

The Reality: Nutrients Are Still Nutrients

This may be a projection from my own relationship with food, but often, I convince myself that modifying foods in certain ways means they "don't count" as healthy anymore. Like if I make a salad and then include bacon and ranch dressing. Or if I top my scrambled eggs with cheese. Or if I swirl a spoonful of Nutella into my vanilla greek yogurt. Of course, the calorie count, fat grams, and/or sugar content changes with these additions. But making these modifications doesn't "cancel out" the nutrients that the original ingredients provide. The lettuce still provides vitamin A. The eggs still provide choline. The yogurt still offers calcium and vitamin D. Making a "healthy food" more desirable doesn't eliminate its nutrients.

This provides peace of mind when I deal with my own picky-eater kid. Would it be great if he'd eat grilled shrimp instead of only accepting fried popcorn shrimp? Yes! But he's still getting protein, omega-3 fatty acids, and vitamin B_{12} from shrimp, and that's a win. Would it be great if he'd eat carrots without drowning them in dressing? Of course! But he's still getting vitamin A (beta-carotene) either way. Would it be ideal if he'd eat french toast without the syrup? Sure—but he's going to get fiber from the bread and protein from the egg even if he covers it with syrup. I'm not going to stress about it, because I know that when we repeatedly expose children to nutrient-rich foods, while doing what we can to enhance a food's palatability (different methods of cooking, seasoning, etc.), we increase our chances that our children will eventually accept them. Let's hope one day he will!

When to Get Help

If your baby is averse to solid foods, will not eat or try entire categories of foods, or is failing to gain weight or reach developmental milestones, please consult with your pediatrician. They may refer your child to feeding therapy, which can be an excellent tool to help expand their palate and evaluate for any oral motor issues that may be contributing to their struggles. Remember, seeking help when you need it is wisdom, not failure!

In a perfect world, our kids would eat what we put in front of them, and what we put in front of them would be well rounded and homemade. If you're able to meet this goal for you and your family each day, that's awesome! I'm often not, and there are a million reasons unique to me, my family, and my circumstances as to why. When I fall short of what I'd like our food situation to be, I don't let myself dwell on it, because I know *fed is best*. I also know I'll get another three chances to try again tomorrow, and another three the day after that, and the day after that.

Fed is best, even when you're outside of the baby stage.

20

Cups, Up! Introducing a Cup

Did you know the American Academy of Pediatrics recommends introducing your baby to a cup when they start eating solids at around six months old? This often catches parents by surprise! In some cases, babies have just gotten the hang of a bottle at that age (if they were primarily breastfed for the first half of their first year). It can feel too early to start messing with cups, but like we discussed with introducing solids, the goal here is exposure and practice at this age, not for your baby to consume the bulk of their liquids from a cup.

What Kind of Cup?

As wild as it sounds, some experts recommend starting with a small open cup. That's right! Rather than using a hard-spouted sippy cup alone, as has been common in past generations, the suggestion is to introduce other types of cups to provide opportunities for your child to learn and develop new, necessary skills. There are also concerns that hard-spouted sippy cups may cause challenges with oral and facial development, although this hasn't been proven.

To use an open cup, the parent or caregiver will hold and tip the cup to the baby's mouth, allowing only a tiny volume of liquid to fall into the mouth to start. Parents can place their hands over their baby's hands, if desired, to help their baby learn the motion of lifting, tilting, drinking, and setting the cup back down! Drinking from a cup requires a different swallowing pattern from a bottle, and offering small, controlled sips can help your baby acclimate to this new skill. If you want to try this method, you can find many varieties of "open training cups" in both silicone and other materials on Amazon or in stores. But you may not even have to purchase something new—a paper medicine cup or shot glass (filled with an appropriate liquid, of course) can get the job done.

If the idea of an open cup sounds horrible (I get it—it's an opportunity for a big, wet mess!), a straw cup is another good option. These cups tend to require a strong suck to pull the liquid through the straw so that they remain "spill-proof" if the baby accidentally—or purposefully—turns the cup over or bangs it on the table. Straw cups can take a bit of time for your baby to get the hang of. Be sure to check the Quick Tip on using a capped straw to get them started!

Another cup that some parents prefer is called a 360 cup. These cups have a lid, making them relatively spill-proof, while still allowing babies to sip from the rim of the cup. For a baby who understands the mechanics of sipping from an open cup, a 360 cup can be a good option to take on the go when you want to reduce the risk of spills.

The ubiquitous sippy cup, also known as a *spout cup*, has fallen out of favor with some parents in recent years. You may find social media posts that discuss the harms of hard-spouted sippy cups for oral development. But as it stands now, a variety of cups are recommended to be introduced—and it's unlikely, based on current knowledge, that your baby will have issues with this assortment-type approach, even if it occasionally includes a spouted cup. Just like you and I can take sips from a straw in a cup at a restaurant, an open cup at home, and a hard-spouted water bottle while on-the-go, offering your baby a variety of cups helps them practice new skills to support their development. Use hard-spouted sippy cups in moderation while other types of cups are also introduced. These cups can be used occasionally but are not recommended as the primary type of cup you offer to your baby or young toddler.

What's in the Cup?

To start, very little! Especially with an open cup, you'll want to limit volume to one or two tablespoons until your baby learns how to manage the flow of liquid. As they become more proficient, the volume in the cup can increase! If you're using a spill-free cup, such as a straw cup, 360 cup, or sippy cup, you can start with two to four ounces of liquid.

It may help to start by offering breast milk or formula in your baby's cup so they associate this new tool with drinking familiar liquids, just like they do with bottles. Some babies, however, want nothing to do with their milk in a cup, and parents may have better success when offering water. This is fine! The Dietary Guidelines for Americans recommend infants between six and twelve months have small amounts of water (no more than four to eight ounces per day). In these months, a substantial amount of nutrition and hydration must continue to come from breast milk or formula—we don't want to fill our baby's belly with water to the point that they're not hungry for their formula or breast milk!

Outside of pediatrician recommendations for addressing constipation—frequently prune or pear juice—fruit juices and other sweetened beverages are not recommended for infants or toddlers under twelve months of age. Keep bottles and cups focused on water and milk during their first two years: breast milk or formula until twelve months, followed by whole cow's milk (or breast milk for as long as you desire) from twelve months to twenty-four months. Plant-based milk alternatives should not be used in the first twelve months as a replacement for breast milk or formula, although unsweetened versions may be used in the second year of life in small amounts.

Why Can't We Stick with Bottles and Offer Water That Way?

Introducing a cup between six to nine months is important because it sets the foundation for weaning from bottles entirely between twelve to eighteen months, as is the AAP's recommendation. When I relay this to parents, I often hear some variation of this question:

Why is it that breastfeeding moms are encouraged to keep nursing until age two or beyond, while formula feeding moms are told to quit the bottle after the first year? The bottle isn't just nutrition for my baby—it's comfort!

The answer brings us back to the (sometimes uncomfortable) truth that while formula and bottles are modeled after breast milk and the breast, they aren't a perfect substitute. Given this, the benefits of extended breastfeeding don't translate to extended formula or bottle feeding. Here's why:

First, a silicone or latex nipple doesn't function in a baby's mouth the same way a human nipple does. A human nipple is malleable, forming to the shape of baby's mouth and palate. With a bottle nipple, the opposite is true—the baby's mouth has to form around the fixed shape. Extended bottle feeding can prevent oral motor skills from developing properly and can also impact how baby teeth descend and position themselves.

Second, the components of formula are able to be sourced from food when your baby reaches their first birthday and is eating a wide variety of table foods. Breast milk, on the other hand, continues to offer bioactive components (like hormones, antibodies, and stem cells) that cannot be found in dietary foods. Given this, breastfeeding offers continued benefits—even for a toddler eating a well-rounded diet—in a way that formula does not. But even breastfed babies need important nutrients, like iron and zinc, from solid foods starting at around six months of age.

The challenges of dropping the bottle don't have to be a source of shame or guilt for those of us who don't have breast milk to offer our toddler! Instead, these reasons are simply the rationale for why continuing to breastfeed makes sense for some families in a way that continuing to bottle feed does not. And, the composition of breast milk aside, even if babies consume breast milk from a bottle, they, too, are encouraged to transition to a cup.

Given this knowledge about why it's important to quit the bottle after the first birthday (and don't worry, we'll cover the how in the coming chapters), we can work backward to understand why we should introduce a cup around six months, even if it feels early. Because the only way to have a proficient toddler who doesn't douse themselves every time they use a cup is to give your baby between now and then to practice.

Quick Tip:
The Capped Straw Strategy

If you've decided to use a straw cup with your baby, the next question quickly becomes obvious: How the heck do you get your baby to suck from a straw? Sucking from a straw requires a different set of skills than sucking from a nipple, and after months of associating a nipple with sucking, many babies look at a straw and have no idea what the heck it is, much less how to use it. You can help your baby learn using a strategy I call *the capped straw*.

At some point, you've likely noticed that if you place a finger or thumb over the top of a straw while it's placed in a drink, you can lift up the straw without the liquid falling out of the bottom. My husband, who's an engineer, says this is due to air pressure—something about creating a low-pressure situation inside the straw that causes pressure from outside the straw to push up, thus preventing the liquid from spilling. In any case, it works.

We can use this trick to help our babies learn that straws are for drinking! Fill a regular drinking glass with water and find a straw—plastic, silicone, or metal, whatever you have on hand. Dip it in the cup, and then cap it with a finger on the top to trap the water inside. Then bring the straw to your baby's mouth. Once your baby has it inside their mouth, remove your finger from the top just a smidge so a bit of water can escape. We want the baby to realize, "Oh! This is a tool for liquids. It's not a bottle, but I can also get liquids this way."

As they start to suck on the straw, provide a bit more water. We want to reward them with water for sucking! This is how they learn that the way to get water from the straw is to suck. You don't want to let all the water fall into your baby's mouth without sucking, as this doesn't teach the association. We want them to learn the cause and effect: "I suck on this thing and I get water." After a few days of practice, many babies will get the hang of this and you can start providing water in their own straw cup.

I prefer this capped straw method, as it doesn't require any special equipment. If this feels too complicated, some parents prefer to teach their babies how to use a straw using a special squeezable straw cup. The most popular one is called a *honey bear cup* (any brand—there are a ton on Amazon), but any cup that you can squeeze and has a straw will work! The strategy is similar: As your baby sucks on the straw, you reward them with water—this time by squeezing the cup so water is pushed up the straw and into your baby's mouth. This creates the same cause and effect opportunity for your baby to learn that if they suck, water will come out of the straw.

No matter which method you choose, investing a bit of time up front to help your baby learn to use a straw will pay dividends. Once they can drink from a cup on their own, you've earned yourself a bit more time and freedom!

9–12 Months

21

How to Drop a Bottle

Doesn't it feel like the second you figure things out with your baby, a new transition sneaks up on you? I hear you—a baby's first year is marked by constant change. One of the transitions that seems to particularly stress parents is when (and how) to start reducing the number of bottles their baby drinks each day. We know that after the first birthday, table food should become the primary source of nutrition, but what's the process to get there? It's not as complicated—or scary—as you might think!

Gradual Reduction in Number of Feedings over Time

If you plan ahead, you can make this transition slowly over

a few months, removing a bottle from your baby's schedule every few weeks and allowing them to adjust before you drop the next one. I don't suggest waiting until your baby is one to start this process! Starting at nine or ten months allows you the time to gradually reduce the number of bottles your baby is drinking each day—and increase the solids they get at meals and snacks—without having to completely overhaul their schedule all at once. I recommend dropping one bottle every three to four weeks and then transitioning any remaining bottle feedings to cups after the first birthday. This may look like:

- **Nine months old:** four to five bottle feedings per day, with six to eight ounces of formula or breast milk in each

- **Ten months old:** four bottle feedings per day, with six to eight ounces in each

- **Eleven months old:** three bottle feedings per day, with seven to eight ounces in each

- **Twelve months old:** two bottle feedings per day, with eight ounces in each

- **Thirteen months old and beyond:** two cups of milk per day, with eight ounces in each

Even if your total number of bottle feedings per day or volume in each feeding differs from the plan above, the overall strategy remains the same—give your baby a few weeks to adjust each time you drop a bottle before removing the next one!

Maintain Total Volume over Time

As you reduce the *frequency* of bottles, you may find it necessary to increase the *volume* of each one. Remember, follow your baby's cues to understand their hunger and fullness. In general, we want a baby to be drinking about two and a half ounces of infant formula per pound of body weight, and usually not more than around thirty-two ounces of formula each day through the first year! If you reduce bottle frequency from five bottles a day to four, for example, you may want to offer a larger volume in each bottle to make up the difference. As your baby approaches eleven and twelve months, both the volume and frequency should naturally reduce as you offer more solids.

Which Bottles to Drop When?

You can choose where to start when it comes to reducing the number of bottles your baby drinks per day. I tend to find that the following order works well, and I have assigned each category an age range I recommend. Know that you can choose a different order and start removing these bottles at a different age from what's suggested here! You know what works best for your schedule, your needs, and your baby.

- **Nighttime bottles (remove between four and twelve months):** For healthy, full-term infants who are growing well, meeting milestones, and maintaining their growth curve percentiles, eating at night past the four-month mark may be due to habit instead of hunger. When seeking to reduce the number of bottles your baby consumes in each twenty-four-hour period as you approach the first birthday, start by removing any remaining night feedings. If you are unsure how to reduce or remove night feedings, I recommend reaching out to a sleep consultant (or looking into their books, guides, or courses). Keep in mind that there are a variety of methods to curtail night wakings, and you may not need to do formal "sleep training" (often known as the *cry-it-out method*)! It's important to address night feedings first, because when we start to remove daytime bottle feedings, we want our babies to make up for those lost calories during the day—not at night.

- **Mealtime bottles (remove between nine and twelve months):** As your baby joins more meals with the family, simply offer solids when you used to offer a bottle. For example, if you had been offering a bottle first thing in the morning, drop that bottle and offer breakfast instead starting around nine or ten months. If you had been offering a bottle at half past four in the afternoon, skip that bottle and offer dinner at five instead starting around ten months.

- **Random, middle-of-the-day bottles (remove between eleven and twelve months):** After you've removed nighttime bottles and bottles that align with mealtimes, next tackle the random bottles throughout the day. For us, this meant dropping the lingering 10:30 a.m. bottle. In this case, you can offer a snack instead (examples in the next Quick Tip!), or see if your baby can wait until lunch—particularly if they had a big breakfast and lunch is on the earlier side.

- **Pre-nap bottle (switch to a cup at twelve months):** My kids loved to have milk before going to sleep, and since roughly sixteen ounces of milk per day is recommended for ages twelve through twenty-four months, we decided to keep those milk servings before nap and before bed. This meant offering a bottle of formula before their nap through the first birthday and then switching to a cup of milk before naptime after.

- **Pre-bedtime bottle (switch to a cup at twelve months):** Same deal here! This feeding can stay if you prefer. Simply switch to milk and a cup after the first birthday.

The How

Now that you have identified which bottle(s) to drop, let's talk about methods for doing so. You have two choices here!

Method 1: Gradual Reduction in Volume by Day

Some parents prefer to slowly reduce the volume offered over time for the feeding they are trying to drop. For example, if you had previously been giving your baby eight ounces of formula or breast milk each morning, and you want to stop this bottle and offer breakfast instead, you may choose to slowly reduce the feeding from eight ounces to six, then four, then two over a number of days before stopping it altogether.

Method 2: Cold Turkey Removal

If you worry your baby will fuss for more milk if you offer only a portion of what they are used to (using the previous method), you can simply decide to stop offering that bottle feeding. This means one day your baby wakes up and you plop them in the high chair for breakfast instead of offering a morning bottle like you had previously. This can be easier in some cases, as the change of scene sets the stage for a different experience from what they're used to!

Either method is fine, and you may choose a different strategy depending on which bottle you are dropping (morning, mealtime, middle of the day, or pre-sleep). As always, the best strategy is the one that works for you and your baby!

Tips for Successful Removal

If your baby is unhappy about not having a bottle (or the same volume of milk) when you start dropping bottles, there are a few things you can try to help ease the transition. These include offering a snack (more on this in the next chapters!), offering a distraction, and/or changing the environment associated with the feeding. Some of my favorite distractions are singing and dancing, taking a walk, doing tummy time, introducing a captivating toy (one with sounds or lights tends to work well) or making funny faces in a mirror.

With regard to the environment, I suggest not keeping the same routine you've always had and only removing the bottle—it can be acutely obvious to your baby what they're missing! Instead, if you used to start every morning with your baby in a rocking chair with their bottle, transition those snuggles to the couch in a different room with a new blanket or toy.

Stay the Course

Removing bottles from your baby's routine can feel scary, I know. It's a big transition, and it's a total shift in how you structure your daily schedule and how your baby receives their nutrition. With intentional planning and a commitment to consistency (don't revert to bottles if the first day or two feels chaotic—it takes time and practice!), it's possible to shepherd your baby successfully from a bottle-based diet to a food-based diet over time without losing your mind (or burning out your nervous system).

Quick Tip:
The Snack Sub

This tip is called "The Snack Sub," but rest assured, we're talking about what to offer your baby instead of a bottle, not about sub sandwiches (which, I suppose, could be deconstructed to become an appropriate snack for a baby, but it wouldn't be at the top of my list). Parents can be apprehensive when dropping bottles because they're afraid their baby won't eat enough with the reduced volume of formula and may start waking up more (or again) at night due to hunger. My favorite way to combat this worry is to offer an equivalent snack—calorie-wise—when you eliminate a non-mealtime bottle from your baby's schedule.

Nearly all infant formulas for healthy, full-term babies offer around twenty calories per fluid ounce. This makes the math really easy! Simply multiply the number of ounces in the feeding you're dropping by twenty, and that will tell you how many calories your baby was typically consuming during that feeding. A five-ounce bottle is about 100 calories. An eight-ounce bottle is about 160 calories. You get the gist! When dropping a bottle, you can choose to offer a snack with the same number of calories as the bottle you're dropping (or close to it). If your little one has a less typical growth pattern (slow weight gain or rapid weight gain), talk to your pediatrician about this plan before implementing it!

And remember, this is just a place to start to give you, as the parent, peace of mind that you're offering roughly the same amount of energy (i.e., calories) to your baby. Keep in mind that if your child is showing signs of greater hunger (or fullness), let them guide how much they need to eat. Your job is to provide the opportunity and the food, and they can choose if and how much they wish to consume!

Here are a few options of snacks for babies to spark some ideas for what you could serve:

- Cheese and whole grain crackers

- Avocado slices (or smashed avocado spread on toast)

- A smoothie with fruit and greek yogurt or nut butter

- Egg bites

- Pineapple and cottage cheese

- Full-fat yogurt

- Sweet potato (cooked and cut appropriately)

- Black beans (create a mash with some olive oil for more calories and fat)

- Cream cheese on strips of whole wheat bread or toast

- Banana slices (with or without a drizzle of thinned-out nut butter on top)

- Whole grain or legume-based pasta (in shapes that are easy to pick up, like rotini or farfalle!) with butter or olive oil

Keep in mind that toddlers (ages one to three) usually need *fewer* calories per pound of body weight than infants because the rate of growth slows down. I know this is hard to believe since toddlers often exist in a constant state of motion, or so it seems! That said, they still need a balanced eating pattern to support their development. Given this, I recommend focusing on *the snack sub* during the late-infancy period (nine to twelve months) as you drop bottles, and then switching your focus to offering well-balanced meals after the first birthday (still offering snacks as needed). The snack sub can help you, as a parent, feel less stressed about losing the nutrition that comes with a bottle and is a good stepping stone as your child transitions to eating more and more solid foods.

Mom Note

Get the Costco Membership for the Berries Alone (and Other Money-Saving Tips)

A baby will eat you under the table without you even realizing. It can be absolutely shocking how much an older baby or young toddler can eat—in many cases, more than my almost-seven-year-old regularly consumes. He survives mostly on air and french fries. For a lot of parents, transitioning to whole cow's milk after the first birthday can feel like getting a raise at work: no more spending twenty to fifty dollars per can of formula! At the same time, however, the increase in monthly grocery costs now that you have another family member eating table food can be surprising. Here are some of my recommended ways to reduce costs during this transition:

- **Buy in bulk:** Costco may be your new best friend! Club stores like Costco, Sam's, and BJ's offer foods at a fraction of the per-item price of a typical grocery store, and they also feature a wide variety of store-brand options for even cheaper. If you know there are certain foods that your baby eats a lot of—berries, crackers, applesauce pouches—buy them in bulk, especially if it's an item that's shelf-stable with a generous expiration date.

- **Start small, then offer more:** Similar to the top-up bottle trick from earlier in the book, it can be a good idea to offer your baby a smaller portion to start and then increase the amount of food on their plate as they eat through it if they are still hungry.

- **Prevent plates from being dumped:** Using a silicone plate with a suction cup on the bottom can be a great way to ensure that your baby's food doesn't get dumped (in their lap or on the floor) in one easy swipe.

- **Catch food before it hits the ground:** Part of the challenge when it comes to lowering food costs with a baby is that so much of the food you offer can go to waste. It ends up smeared all over their high chair, tangled in their hair, stuck up their nose, thrown on the floor, and more. I can't help with the smearing and the hair, but a few companies now offer a "food catcher" attachment that goes around the legs of your baby's high chair to catch food that's dropped or thrown. As long as you keep this piece of equipment clean (the same way you would a high chair tray!), you can save food that is caught and reoffer it to your baby at the same meal or a future one.

- **Make food for the whole family:** Baby-specific foods—like yogurt melts, teething biscuits, and fruit and veggie pouches—can be convenient, but they're also expensive. Offering your baby the same foods the rest of the family is eating (served in age-appropriate preparations and sizes) can help lower costs. If you missed it, check out the "I'll Have What You're Having" Quick Tip for more on this!

- **Introduce a "no thank you" bowl:** Often, babies throw food they don't want to eat. It can be helpful to place a small plate or bowl (with a suction cup on the bottom, if desired) next to their meal and show them where to place the food they don't want. This takes time and practice to learn, but one day, you're likely to end up with a bowl full of green beans that someone else can eat rather than a floor full of them.

- **Save (and freeze) what you can:** I don't tend to save leftovers for myself if there's less than a full portion still available. But with a baby, even a single leftover broccoli floret can be repurposed! Invest in some small containers, and save everything for the fridge or freezer to offer again later.

- **Focus on nutrient-dense foods that are lower cost:** Beans, eggs, milk, oatmeal, bananas, potatoes, cottage cheese, and peanut butter are just a few foods that pack a big nutritional punch with a reasonably small price tag.

There are many ways to reduce costs—and waste—while feeding an older baby or young toddler, and if you're intentional about it, you very well might save money compared to what you previously spent on formula!

22

Trading Formula for Milk

With part one of the baby-to-toddler drink transition off to a good start (reducing bottles and moving to cups, a.k.a. the *how* for drinking past age one), you're now approaching part two: moving from formula to cow's milk (or another alternative, a.k.a. the *what* for their drinking past age one). You have a lot of options here! Let's go through them.

Types of Milk or "Milk"

- **Cow's milk:** The AAP recommends whole cow's milk for toddlers ages one to two because it contains protein and fat as well as crucial nutrients like vitamin D, vitamin A, and calcium. Growing

toddlers need these! While regular whole milk is
perfectly fine, you can also select a milk option that's
been fortified with other nutrients, such as DHA (an
omega-3 fatty acid) or choline, and/or with prebiotic fiber to support healthy poops. These milks tend
to be advertised with names like "growing years" and
"family first." One cup of whole milk contains about
150 calories, 8 grams of protein, 8 grams of fat, 12
grams of carbohydrates, 310 mg of calcium, and 100
IU (2.5 mcg) vitamin D. You'll want to keep these
details in mind as you evaluate milk alternatives,
if alternatives are important to you or preferred.
Ideally, you want your young toddler's milk to align
as closely with the nutrition offered by whole cow's
milk as possible!

- **Goat's milk:** Goat's milk offers similar nutrition to
  cow's milk in terms of protein (goat's milk is slightly
  lower), lactose (also slightly lower) and fat (nearly
  equivalent if both options are labeled "whole milk").
  Whole goat's milk may be suitable for some toddlers
  who have trouble digesting cow's milk, as goat's milk
  contains predominantly A2 beta-casein proteins
  (compared to A1 beta-casein proteins), although it
  would not be appropriate for a toddler with a medically established cow's milk protein allergy or lactose
  intolerance. Discuss with your pediatrician whether
  goat's milk could be a good option for your little one
  if you'd prefer not to offer cow's milk.

- **Soy milk:** For parents who prefer a plant-based option, the AAP lists fortified soy milk as the only plant-based alternative that is suitable for children since it offers protein, vitamin D, and calcium. If you plan to offer soy milk, choose an unsweetened version to limit how many added sugars your toddler consumes.

- **Pea milk:** This plant-based milk option made with pea protein is newer to the market and has found favor among parents who want to avoid both dairy and soy. Although not recommended by the AAP, some parents use this option. If choosing this kind of milk for your little one, be sure to prioritize a brand that offers nutrients similar to those found in whole cow's milk, which means plenty of fat and protein per serving along with calcium and vitamin D! Be sure to read labels to understand the amount of added sugar that may be present, and opt for an unsweetened pea milk instead of a sweetened product.

- **Oat milk:** This is another new and increasingly popular option for parents who want a plant-based "milk," although it, too, is not recommended by the AAP. If you decide to serve oat milk, as with pea milk, look for a brand that provides enough fat and protein—some brands will offer low-fat and full-fat options just like we see with cow's milk, and full-fat is what you want for your one-year-old! Note that

the fat in oat milk, like pea milk, is primarily from
plant-based oils, as oats do not contain much fat
inherently. You'll also want to be mindful of the
amount of added sugar in oat milk so that you can
help your toddler consume less, so be sure to read
labels. While you're reading labels, also check to see
if the oat milk is fortified with calcium and vitamin
D, just like you'd find present in cow's milk or a fortified soy milk.

- **Toddler formulas:** The AAP does not recommend
  toddler formulas as an alternative to cow's milk,
  largely because they tend to be expensive and many
  of them contain added sugars (beyond the lactose
  sugar content you'd naturally find in dairy milk).
  Some parents may prefer a toddler formula, however,
  as they are shelf-stable (good for traveling) and can
  be more nutrient and calorie dense per serving than
  cow's milk or a plant-based milk alternative. If you
  choose to use a toddler formula, I suggest looking
  for one that contains only lactose for the carbohydrate (if dairy-based) and that offers similar fat and
  protein to whole milk.

- **Other plant-based milks:** While almond milk, rice
  milk, and even hemp milk have become popular
  among adults in recent years, these milks are not
  recommended for toddlers, as most are not nutritionally equivalent, or even close, to whole cow's

milk. However, out of preference, some parents may choose to offer these to their children. If so, be sure to talk to your child's pediatrician about finding and serving alternative food sources for the nutrients that are typically offered by whole milk.

- **No milk at all:** Some parents are choosing to skip milk altogether in favor of sourcing protein, fat, and nutrients from whole foods instead—particularly from other dairy products, such as yogurt and cheese. If you'd prefer to skip milk entirely, talk to your pediatrician about how to ensure your toddler is getting all the nutrients they need from their diet.

How to Introduce a New Milk

Like we've discussed in prior chapters that cover transitions, you have the same two choices here when it comes to starting milk: You can introduce it gradually, phasing in the milk and out the formula over time, or you can simply make a one-to-one swap. Here's how!

The Gradual Transition

Some parents may choose to slowly reduce the amount of formula their baby is taking and help them acclimate to the taste of milk by combining milk in the same bottle or cup as their baby's prepared formula (mix powdered formula with water first as instructed on the back of the container). This may look like starting with six ounces of prepared formula and adding two ounces of milk (in the same bottle or cup) for an eight-ounce total serving for a few days, then four ounces of formula and four ounces of milk for a few days, then two ounces of formula and six ounces of milk for a few days, until you've switched over to entirely eight ounces of milk.

The Cold Turkey Swap

Alternatively, it may be easier to simply stop giving formula and start giving milk, particularly if your baby isn't picky. This can make for a quicker transition and will also give you data much sooner about how your baby is tolerating whatever milk or milk alternative you've chosen to offer.

Temperature Troubles

A common challenge parents don't anticipate when introducing milk is their baby's preference for a certain temperature. If you've been routinely warming your baby's bottles, they likely expect their milk to be warm. If you've been serving room-temperature bottles, a cold glass of milk may be off-putting! If you know your baby is temperature-sensitive, I suggest trying to acclimate your baby to a refrigerated temperature for their formula or breast milk *before* you try to introduce cold milk. Once they accept a cold beverage that we already know they prefer, it is easier to introduce a new beverage in that same cold-from-the-fridge temperature. Alternately, you can choose to continue to warm their milk when you switch from formula (many of us grew up with a warm cup of milk before bed!) or use shelf-stable, individual-size cartons of cow's milk for a room-temperature option.

Don't Go Overboard on Milk!

It's crucial when switching to cow's milk or a milk alternative that you don't simply replace all the formula your baby's been drinking with their new milk. The AAP recommends sixteen ounces of milk per day between one and two years of age, and no more than twenty-four ounces per day. Allowing too much milk per day can result in reduced intake of solid foods (preventing your toddler from receiving the wide variety of nutrients they need) and increased risk of iron deficiency and iron-deficient anemia.

"But if I don't offer milk, my baby won't eat anything!"

I often hear from parents that are highly concerned about reducing their young toddler's milk intake because they know their kiddo doesn't eat many solids, and at least the milk provides calories and some important nutrients. They are worried if they reduce their little one's access to milk, they won't get enough calories or nutrients from solid foods. The issue often becomes a chicken-and-egg cyclical situation—their toddler doesn't eat solids, so the parent provides milk, and then the toddler continues to not eat solids, because they're full from the milk.

While a bit scary, often the solution (for healthy children with no known medical reason to explain their eating challenges) is to reduce your child's access to milk—down to the recommended sixteen ounces per day—and trust that their solids consumption will very likely pick up. Know that this may take a bit of time. Your toddler may cry for milk when you give them a meal! They may eat very little for a few days. With your pediatrician's approval, stick to the plan. Your toddler is resilient, and in all likelihood, they will figure out how to address their hunger with food. As my pediatrician assured me often, "Most kids are very good at not letting themselves lose weight."

If your child has a difficult time with solids, does not increase their eating after a few days of reduced milk consumption, or begins to lose weight, please consult with their doctor. They may recommend further evaluation or a referral to feeding therapy, which can be very helpful in navigating challenges during the bottles-to-cups and formula-to-food transition.

Bonus Note: Managing Constipation Post-Milk Introduction

Don't be surprised if you notice firmer, less frequent stools once you switch from formula or breast milk to cow's milk. This is common! Excess dairy consumption is known to contribute to constipation. If you find yourself in this situation, here are some tips to try to address it:

- Reduce overall milk and dairy consumption.

- Ensure your little one is drinking enough water (one to four cups a day is recommended between one and two years of age).

- Introduce *P* fruits like pears, prunes, and papayas, since these offer fiber like many other fruits.

- Make sure you're offering foods with fiber—like beans, broccoli, berries, and (whole grain) breads, sometimes called *B* foods, in addition to other fruits, vegetables, and whole grains that offer fiber.

- Discuss with your child's pediatrician whether a pre- and probiotic supplement may make sense. Research is mixed on whether these supplements support softer stool texture, but some parents may find they help.

If constipation continues, consult with your child's pediatrician to assess for other explanations and discuss treatment options.

Quick Tip:
The Milk Cup

You should know up front that this tip has no formal research basis to support what I'm about to say. This suggestion is based solely on my experiences and those of the people around me, including my sister and sisters-in-law, which provides a sample size of eleven babies in eight years (yes, it's wild when we all get together and *so very loud*). If anecdotal evidence doesn't work for you, feel free to skip! I find, however, that it can be helpful to hear what worked for others, even if it's based on a hunch.

When transitioning from formula or breast milk to cow's milk (or a milk alternative), and also from bottles to cups, it can be helpful to identify a certain cup as *the milk cup*. We know that babies can get attached to their bottles—it becomes a comfort item and in some cases creates a sleep association. Babies see the bottle and know what to expect: *I'm going to get milk, and then I'm going to take a nap.* The bottle itself can be a cue. As we transition away from bottles, swapping in another cup that your baby can associate with milk and attach expectations to can help them adjust.

Let's put this in an adult context. Have you ever expected water, only to take a drink from your glass to discover it's Sprite? It's disconcerting, even if you like Sprite! Do you have a preferred coffee cup that you use every morning, or a special cup you only use for certain purposes or occasions? I have a glass cup in the shape of a boot that I inherited from my grandmother, and it comes with a million positive memories. I pick that cup—even today—when I have something to celebrate. It's natural to want to know what's in a cup before we drink—and to create associations with certain cups!

Given this, I suggest having a designated cup for

your baby's milk (or a few in the same style so you're not washing the same one several times a day) that's different from their water cups. This creates predictability for them, and predictability can help ease stress for everyone.

Some of you may be rolling your eyes and wondering if this is too much work or may create neurosis around cups. Keep in mind that this doesn't have to last forever! By late toddlerhood and in the preschool years, my kids didn't care at all what cups were used for what purpose (though they did care about the color—give a green cup to a kid who wants a blue cup at your own risk). In early toddlerhood, though, when little ones can't communicate very effectively and are still learning that there's a whole world out there of different flavors and textures, keeping milk to a predictable cup can be helpful.

23

Quitting the Bottle Altogether

Let's say you've been successful in reducing the number of bottles your baby is drinking each day over the course of several weeks and months. Now you're down to one or two bottles a day. If I had to guess, the last remaining bottle your baby takes is a pre-bedtime bottle. This one can be the very hardest to quit, as it's often ingrained in an established routine that is working for everyone—baby's happy, parents are happy, baby sleeps well. Often, parents are hesitant to mess with this: If it ain't broke, don't fix it, right? In this chapter, we'll cover the recommended age to stop the last bottle, why it's recommended, and different methods for making this transition as easy as possible (so you can hopefully avoid a significant disruption of your bedtime routine).

When to Stop Bottles

The AAP, the American Academy of Pediatric Dentistry, and the USDA all have recommendations for when to discontinue bottle use, ranging from twelve months to eighteen months. Before age one, when breast milk or formula is your child's primary source of nutrition, bottles are a crucial piece of equipment to ensure adequate consumption of nutrients. After age one, however, when your baby's primary nutrition should come from solid foods, bottles no longer serve the same important function. It can give parents whiplash how quickly bottles switch from "the reason my baby is thriving" to "the creator of possible negative consequences." Understanding why these organizations recommend stopping bottles by a year and a half can help with this whiplash!

Why It's Important to Stop Bottles

We briefly discussed in chapter 20 that bottle nipples, made of silicone or latex, do not function in a baby's mouth the same way a human nipple does. They are less malleable, sit in a different position in the mouth, and require different muscle coordination to use. Used long-term, this can prevent proper tooth alignment and speech development in toddlerhood. Additionally, using bottles beyond infancy has been shown to increase the risk of certain outcomes, such as dental decay (especially when bottles are given frequently or at night), iron deficiency, and it is even a risk factor for obesity. I don't say this to scare you! *It's okay if it takes some time to transition your baby off their last bottle.* Instead, use this knowledge as a motivator to do the hard work of eliminating the bottle, knowing your baby will benefit from it.

Methods for Quitting That Last Bottle

There are several ways you can approach removing the final bottle from your baby's routine. This transition can feel harder than the others—for both parent(s) and baby— because it closes the door on an important chapter of your child's feeding journey. Additionally, older babies and young toddlers tend to have stronger feelings about giving up the bottle than they may have had when you started removing other bottles earlier in life. The older the child, the more opinions they tend to have! Here are some of my favorite options for getting rid of the last bottle:

- **Switch to a cup:** This method is the most straightforward, and it follows the same instructions you're familiar with from dropping other bottles. When it comes time for your baby's typical bottle feeding, offer their milk (formula or breast milk under age one; whole cow's milk or an alternative if they're past twelve months) in a cup instead. Your little one can choose whether to drink it or not, but you've given them the option!

- **Dilute the milk:** One way to get your baby to stop wanting their bottle is to make it less enticing. Some parents choose to do this by diluting the milk over the course of days or weeks until it's largely water, as this reduces their baby's interest in it. Simultaneously, you can offer a full, undiluted serving of milk in a cup so that if your baby is frustrated by the option in the bottle, they can get what they want by choosing the cup! If your baby typically drinks eight ounces of milk in their bottle, start by offering a bottle with six ounces of milk and two ounces of water. A few days later, make it four ounces of milk with four ounces of water. By the time it's two ounces of milk and six ounces of water, the likelihood that your baby will want to drink it is much lower. Once the bottle no longer provides what they're looking for, many babies won't want it anymore.

- **Bottle fairy:** Taking a more benevolent approach, this method instructs that you involve your child in packing up all their bottles and then leaving them out for "the bottle fairy" to take away to give to a baby—reinforcing that babies are who bottles are meant for. Some parents choose to leave a small gift "from the bottle fairy" in place of the bottles once they have been "picked up." This method tends to work better for toddlers who can understand and will buy into this make-believe scenario.

- **Cold turkey:** If all these strategies feel like too much, you can choose to remove the last bottle without any fanfare. Simply decide the day that you won't offer it anymore. This may result in more fussing than the other methods but can result in a quicker outcome.

Be Consistent

It's common knowledge that parents don't like to hear their baby cry. For our species' survival, it's a biological imperative that we respond to our babies' cries, and this creates a strong desire to "fix" whatever causes our babies distress. In infancy, this is important! Cries alert us to hunger or other discomforts that need our attention.

In toddlerhood, we have to evaluate whether a cry needs intervention, and in some cases, we must actively choose *not* to intervene if what's causing our kiddo(s) to cry is important for their development, health, or safety. For example, if your child cries every time you put them in the car seat, it's not an option, legally, to let them ride without a car seat to prevent them from crying. We know, in this example, that keeping them safe is more important than making sure they don't get upset.

The same principle applies here. Your baby may cry when you remove their final bottle. This is tough to watch, and you may be tempted to give in and offer a bottle again so they stop being sad. I encourage you to stay strong! Your baby is resilient, and they can learn to exist happily without their bottle if we give them the gift of practice—and this means being consistent in not offering it to them, even if they're mad about it. This transition might feel painful for both the child and the parent, but it can serve as a good opportunity to practice coping skills *and* prioritize what's best for your child's development over their (fleeting) feelings.

Maintaining Closeness and Comfort Post-Bottle

For some parents, it's harder for *them* to give up the last bottle than it is for the baby. The bottle can become a tangible symbol of comfort and care for the parent, and removing the bottle symbolizes the true end of their baby's babyhood. It's a big deal! In this case, I encourage you to remember that removing the bottle itself doesn't mean you have to lose everything bottle feeding provided: time throughout the day to stop and rest with your baby, the opportunity to hold your baby close, periods of prolonged eye contact, and the weight of a warm, sleepy little one in your arms.

You can continue these moments with a cup in place of a bottle, or build them into your schedule outside of mealtimes. You can rock your baby, sing to your baby, and do skin to skin with your baby outside of feeding times! Continuing these breaks for connection throughout the day can benefit both the parent and the baby during the transition away from the bottle, because so much of the comfort of feeding your baby was never about the bottle or milk—it was about the closeness. And this, thankfully, doesn't have to end when the bottle does!

Mom Note
Releasing Control

I'm nearly ten years into my motherhood journey, and while I've learned a lot, I don't pretend to have it all figured out.

There are very few things I know for sure, but this is one of them: Parenthood is marked by the never-ending process of releasing control. Every month—and then year—that passes means more independence for your kiddo and less control for you.

When they're a newborn, you control *everything*:

- What they wear.

- What they eat.

- When they eat.

- When they nap.

- Who they interact with.

- Where they go.

- What they play with.

- Et cetera, et cetera, et cetera.

As they age, more and more of these things (and then all the things, really) shift from your responsibility to theirs. Before you know it, they will want to decide what to wear. They will decide to stop napping, even if you put them in their crib or in their room to rest. They will decide what toys to play with and which toys they hate. Even later, they will decide where to go and with whom. Eventually, they'll make decisions they don't even tell you about, like applying to and then committing to a college you'd never even heard them mention because their high school boyfriend got accepted there (sorry, Mom).

Parenthood is the slow, painful journey of releasing control.

Right about now, you're probably thinking, *Geez, Mallory—what a way to dampen the mood, talking about my baby leaving the nest one day when I'm just celebrating their first birthday.* I know, your child's growing independence is a bittersweet truth, and it likely feels much too soon to be thinking about long-term. But it's important, because some of the very first ways you'll need to release control with your baby happen around twelve months, and they center around eating. And how you approach this release can set a foundation for how you approach *all* the releases to come.

Releasing control is a muscle you'll need to learn to flex, and it starts now.

For an entire year, you have decided both what your baby is eating (formula, breast milk, solids) and when. Of course, they've decided whether to eat and how much, but on the whole, *feeding* has fallen squarely under your jurisdiction. Most likely, your baby has eaten whatever you offered in their bottle, at the amount offered (most of the time). This has likely provided you with assurance that they are getting the nutrients and calories they need.

With the switch to solid foods and away from formula and bottles, there's no such assurance. Some days, you will feel like your toddler has eaten way too much and is bound to throw it all up. Other days, you'll wonder whether they've had a vegetable all week, and whether french fries count (they do; see "'Fed Is Best' Applies to Table Food, Too!"). Occasionally, you may worry you've messed up their eating habits for life. Rarely, you'll think about whether you'd do something differently if you could go back and redo it—even though you can't. It's not an easy thing for a lot of us, mentally and emotionally, to let go of food control with our little ones.

Here's what you should try to remember: Your new toddler is so much more resilient than you think, and their body knows what they need. If they only eat bread for a day? They'll be fine. If they eat five servings of watermelon? Totally okay (but watch out for the poops). The best thing we can do to set our kids up for a healthy relationship with food is to offer a wide variety and let them eat what they want to eat (and how much of it they want to eat).

If you're like me, you will likely feel tempted to barter (i.e., "If you eat one bite of broccoli, you can have more strawberries!"). You may find yourself wanting to withhold their preferred food until the end of the meal so they have to eat the "healthy stuff" first. You might itch to encourage them to clear their plate, or not let them leave the table until they've finished their milk. A lot of us grew up with these experiences, and I will readily admit I sometimes fall into these patterns even now. But still I encourage you: Try to release your grip of control on whether—and how much—your little one eats now that they're past age one. You might drive yourself crazy if you don't. Remember:

- Your job is to decide what to serve and when.

- Their job is to decide whether to eat and how much.

If you can lean in here and let go of control, you may quickly find that it all turns out okay. This feedback then encourages and bolsters you for the next time you have to release control (like for potty training—oof). This becomes the pattern, an undulation, of your experience in parenthood. We release control with gritted teeth, and our kid shows us they're capable. We release more control with gritted teeth, and they show us they're capable again. More to the point: This is how they *become* capable—by figuring things out for themselves, and often by failing first. And meanwhile, we grit our teeth harder. On the off chance they aren't capable? Then we get them whatever external support they need.

I'd like to tell you that releasing control becomes easier over time. It doesn't. In fact, it may become harder; as your kid ages, the stakes become higher. And while it doesn't get easier, with time and practice, you will get better at it.

My encouragement to you is to start now, with feeding, even though it feels too early and like their brains are still much too immature to decide whether they've had enough to eat. Start practicing now anyway. It'll serve you both for years to come.

24

Celebrating Yourself

You did it! You made it through (what may have been) one of the most challenging years you've ever had. You look down at your baby and marvel at how much they've changed: They might have more hair now, they might be saying a few words, they might be crawling or walking, they might be eating real foods and actually playing with toys. Just a few months ago, these things were different. They have skills now they simply did not have when the year started.

And you, parent of the year, do, too.

Your baby will likely receive a lot of celebration as they reach their first birthday. Friends, neighbors, grandparents, coworkers, and more may want to join in. There might be cake to smash and then smear all over their sweet little face, presents to unwrap, and a big-kid car seat to install. It's easy and oh so fun to celebrate our babies and how much they've grown!

It can be a lot harder to celebrate ourselves.

When you arrive at this milestone, I want you to take a few minutes (seriously, no less than ten!) and celebrate how far *you've* come this year:

- You kept your baby fed, no matter how hard the journey has been.

- You navigated approximately 378 different transitions.

- You dealt with *so many* bodily fluids.

- You survived on little sleep.

- You learned entirely new skills that you had no prior experience with and then implemented them.

- You learned your baby's likes and dislikes.

- You learned how to comfort your baby.

- You kept yourself fed and showered and functioning (even imperfectly).

- You rocked, and swayed, and held your baby for hundreds (thousands?) of hours.

- You communicated care for your family with your words and actions, day in and day out.

- You set the foundation for your child to thrive, for whatever that may look like for them.

- You didn't give up when things were difficult—even exceptionally so. (And don't tell me you did "give up" because you quit breastfeeding. You didn't give up—*you pivoted*. You worked every day to keep your baby fed. You didn't run away from the challenge. You pushed through it, and that's a win.)

- You learned a whole lot about yourself and what's important to you and what can take a back seat.

- You likely learned a lot about your relationships (with your family of origin, a partner, and/or friends).

- You woke up every single day and did the damn thing—whatever it was that needed to be done.

- _____

- _____

- _____

I left three lines here for you to fill in with things you're especially proud of this year. If you're anything like I am, your default may be to stew over everything you think you did "wrong." Are there people out there who don't? I certainly wouldn't know. Whether you're a stewer or celebrator, take a minute and jot down what you've done, learned, or changed this year that makes you feel proud. You deserve to be acknowledged for the effort, even if you're the one doing the acknowledging.

My mom has always said mothers should be celebrated on birthdays, not just kids. Most years, she sends my twin sister and me a text on our birthday that essentially says, "You're welcome for all my hard work." For a long time, this felt silly and self-gratifying, but now that I'm a parent, I get it. When a kid has a birthday, so much of what they've gained in the past year is a direct result of the effort of the people in their lives (not just parents but also teachers, nannies, family members, friends). It's worth celebrating these people, too, for what they've learned and the skills they've acquired.

Many of your baby's accomplishments only exist because of the environment *you* created for them. That's worth celebrating.

So take yourself out to dinner. Buy a balloon and your favorite flowers at the store. Wear the nice outfit from your closet that you've wondered if you'd ever wear again now that you spend most of your time covered in snot and food residues. Or, if you have a partner or friend who can help out with bedtime, treat yourself to a night off and eat Oreos and scroll social media and watch your favorite trashy TV. Whatever feels celebratory to you!

What you did this year *is no small thing*. It's a huge thing, and it will benefit your baby for the rest of their life. Take a moment to feel good about that.

You did it. You really, truly did it.

Now on to year two!

25

Society Hates a Happy Mom
(Be One Anyway)

When my first baby finished her formula journey, I remember thinking how grateful I was to be out of the pressure cooker of the "breast is best" world around me. We lived through the gauntlet of opinions, shame, judgment, and disappointment hurled by so many different people—well-meaning nurses at the hospital, concerned family members, strangers on the internet, old ladies in the grocery store—and we survived. The drama was *done*.

That's really what I thought.

I quickly discovered, as you may have, that drama based on differing opinions and beliefs in the parenting world is *never* done. Unless you live off the grid, there is always someone ready to tell you that whatever you're doing is wrong and that your kid will suffer because of it. There always will be. Some people make their living—and others make themselves feel important—by tearing others down.

Here's where you have a secret advantage: This first year with your baby, you learned how to prioritize what works for you and your family. You ignored the noise to feed your baby the way you wanted to, or had to, no matter the voices and opinions from outside your home. You have experience guarding your heart and mind from people and recommendations that don't serve you and your particular circumstances. Not everyone has this! Working through a challenging feeding journey—or one you didn't expect—means you've developed a muscle for making your own way, regardless of the popular narrative.

This ability—to do things the way you need to do them, without guilt or shame—is the secret to being a happy mom.

(Well, one of them. A living wage for all, affordable childcare, and paid parental leave would also help. Give me uninterrupted sleep, time to read a book in a quiet house, plus a bag of Doritos if you want to seal the deal.)

Vocally self-assured, happy moms tend to be villainized in our culture. We're called selfish. We're accused of not loving our kids enough or caring more about ourselves (or our careers, or our looks, or our status) than our kids. More than one person on the internet has said that if I wasn't willing to sacrifice *everything* for my kids, including my physical and mental health, I never should have had them.

How did we get here? Why is the most common definition of a "good mom" one who has stripped herself down to the bone in service of others and who has nothing left for herself?

Let's challenge this narrative.

The motherhood I want for my daughter someday (if she chooses to have kids) doesn't look like endless self-sacrifice on the altar of what society thinks is "best." I want her to make the choices that are right for her, and I want her to not feel bad about it! Because I know she is smart and capable of evaluating what her family needs and making the right calls. I want her to have a life outside of her kids—a meaningful career if she wants one, strong friendships, hobbies, some free time. I want her to know she doesn't have to listen to the opinions of others about her mothering, because she's the only one who knows the truth about all she does, how much she cares, and what her family needs.

If I want that kind of motherhood for my daughter someday—and just as important, if I want my son to know this is what motherhood should look like, not a woman killing herself for everyone else's benefit—*I need to model it*. I want these things for my daughter because I care about her so much. Modeling it means caring about myself—and my motherhood, too.

My challenge for you is to be the mom you want or need to be, even if it's outside the scope of "good" or "right" or "best" according to some (providing your decisions are safe, of course).

It won't just benefit you and your kid(s). If I've learned anything in my years as The Formula Mom, it's this:

Living in freedom for yourself gives others courage and permission to do the same.

So go out there and be a confident, happy mom. Take the skills you learned this year about tuning out the opinions of people who aren't living your same circumstances and apply them to other areas of your life, too. Refuse to feel bad about the ways your journey looks different from others'. When we step into confidence knowing we're doing our best for our kids—even if it's not the "best" we see hung up in flashing lights on social media—everyone benefits.

You can do it. I know you can because you just proved it with your baby's feeding journey. Take this experience and let it empower you as you go forward in your parenting, because while the hard choices don't stop, neither does a strong parent. And that, my friend, is you.

Additional Resources

While I did my best to make this book as comprehensive as possible, I am confident you will have questions during your baby's first year (feeding journey and otherwise!) that this book doesn't address. Here are a few additional resources for high-quality, evidence-based information about infant feeding and/or formula:

- Your child's pediatrician! They know you and your child best. I always suggest starting here with your questions.

- HealthyChildren.org (www.healthychildren.org): This is the American Academy of Pediatrics' public-facing website. This site is full of information covering all sorts of topics—feeding, developmental milestones, illness, what's normal/what's not, and so much more!

- *Feed the Baby: An Inclusive Guide to Nursing, Bottle-Feeding, and Everything in Between* by Victoria Facelli, IBCLC. Victoria is a friend and colleague, and she is the most formula-friendly and inclusive lactation consultant I've ever known! If you have

breastfeeding questions, combo feeding questions,
or questions about tube feeding or other feeding
methods, this book is a fantastic resource.

- *The Pediatrician's Guide to Feeding Babies and Toddlers: Practical Answers to Your Questions on Nutrition, Starting Solids, Allergies, Picky Eating, and More (for Parents, by Parents)* by Anthony Porto, MD, and Dina DiMaggio, MD. I'm also lucky to call Dina and Anthony friends and colleagues! Both are practicing clinicians, infant feeding researchers, and AAP spokespeople. Their book offers comprehensive education for infant feeding and beyond.

- *Solid Starts for Babies: How to Introduce Solid Food and Raise a Happy Eater* by Solid Starts. You can also find education at @solidstarts on social media, www.solidstarts.com, and the Solid Starts app! The entire team at Solid Starts is incredible and includes pediatricians, dietitians, occupational therapists, feeding and swallowing specialists, and a speech-language pathologist who specializes in infant and toddler feeding. Solid Starts is my go-to resource for all things (as you may have guessed!) starting solids.

- The Food and Drug Administration (www.fda .gov) provides updates on infant formula regulation, safety, and recalls. This is the best place to search

for up-to-date information on what's happening
industry-wide from a regulatory perspective.

These are just a few of the many incredible resources that
exist to support parents in feeding their infants. Because I
know how overwhelming it can be to try to sort through endless resources and information, I'll leave it at this!

Acknowledgments

They say it takes a village to raise a child, and it also takes a village to write, publish, and market a book! As tempted as I am to call this book my (third) baby, it belongs not just to me but to so many wonderful people who helped my thoughts and words become the finished product you hold today.

Wendy Sherman and Callie Deitrick—you saw my vision from day one (manifested it, even!) and found the perfect home for my work with a dream imprint. Thank you for being patient with me, pushing me, and shepherding me on this journey. I couldn't ask for better agents.

Sam Weiner, thank you for taking a chance on *Bottle Service* even though nothing like it existed in the market to show proof of concept. Your edits made it stronger, and I am thrilled it was a resource for your own newborn feeding journey! You're the best person who could've acquired and championed this book.

Tori Schmitt, MS, RDN, LD, you are the greatest-of-all-time fact-checker and reference wrangler. This book would be a hot mess of opinions, outdated recommendations, and mismatched endnotes if it weren't for your diligent care with the manuscript. Thank you for sharing your expertise and for your graciousness with both my words and my intent.

Gina Navaroli, Lauren Morino, Francesca Carlos, Jenny

Carrow, Carah Gedeon, and the entire Simon Element team, you have made this book come to life in ways I couldn't have dreamed. From the cover design, to getting it into bookstores, to the many incredible marketing and publicity opportunities, y'all are the best of the best.

Laura Modi, Kim Chappell, Sara Holman, and the Bobbie fam, you saw the magic in my work first, and I am forever grateful for the ways you've supported my career both inside and outside of Bobbie. This book wouldn't exist without your encouragement. An additional shout-out to Alex, Shira, and Paige—your friendship kept me going during the writing process. Thank you for listening to my whining and encouraging my work!

William Warren, my brother-in-law, who told me for years I should write a formula book proposal and query it. You were right. Thank you as well for the amazing illustrations featured in chapter 8!

Nancy Morse, the original formula mom (a.k.a. *my* mom), who is featured throughout this work with all kinds of wisdom I'm blessed to receive daily. I'm sorry we didn't go with one of your title suggestions for this book. Thank you for modeling what it means to love and care for your kids without driving yourself crazy to meet someone else's standards. You give the best advice. And Alan Morse, my dad, who also contributed wisdom to these pages and who convinced me to sign with Simon Element for this book. You also give the best advice.

For my twinny—my sister, Monica Warren—who saw me in the throes of postpartum depression, asked me the hard questions about the support I needed, shared her breast milk when mine was MIA before I started formula, made content for me for The Formula Mom, and who continues to deal with people stopping her on the street several times a year thinking she's me, and who is otherwise the absolute best friend, confidante, and supporter—I love doing motherhood with you. I don't know how people live who don't have a twin (sorry to the rest of you).

Tyler, my husband and biggest fan, who never misses an opportunity to tell anyone who will listen how impressive his wife is. I've said it before and I'll say it forever—thank you for never once treating my impulsive, wild ideas as silly. Whether I'm starting an Instagram account during COVID lockdown, or writing a rom-com, or flying to Spain for a three-day birthday trip, your support emboldens and empowers me, and I'm so much better for it. Thank you for believing in me even when you don't understand what I'm trying to do or why, and especially when I don't believe in myself. I got the best one!

Sweet T, my best girl and the catalyst for The Formula Mom, this work, and all the best things I've ever done. Being your mom has pushed me in ways I didn't realize I needed. You get the learning-as-I-go version of my motherhood, and you are so gracious as I (and we) continue to figure out what the heck we're doing together. I know my journey-to-formula story is also your newborn story, and I don't take for granted that you let me share it. I love you infinitely.

Mr. Dude, the boy who healed my postpartum heartache and helped me come into my own choices around newborn feeding. You are exactly what our family needed, then and now, and it is a gift to be your mom. Thank you for sharing me with my computer much more than normal these past few years as I was getting these words on the page. I love you to the moon.

My other family, IRL friends, coworkers, influencer friends, and anyone else I'm surely missing, I appreciate you.

To the followers, fans, and friends of The Formula Mom— it has been the privilege of my life supporting you, listening to your stories, helping you through your challenges, and championing your wins. Thank you for creating a space with me on the Wild West internet where we can be authentic and discuss the difficult realities of feeding a baby—and how we might make it easier. The last six years of my life, and all the opportunities contained within, have only been possible because of you. Thank you.

For the new mom (or dad) reading this, thank you for picking up this book and investing in yourself and your baby in this small way. You are doing the thing, and I know it's so hard some days, but you're figuring it out. I'm proud of you! I know it's rude to ask a new parent to do something (y'all have enough on your plate!), but I'd be so grateful if you could share the word about this book with your friends, neighbors, online mom groups, pediatrician, and anyone else you think could benefit. I'll refrain from asking you to leave a review of the book, but if you want to, I'd love you forever.

References

Mom Note: I See You, Because I've Been There

4 not *exclusively breastfeeding*: *Breastfeeding Report Card: United States, 2022* (Centers for Disease Control and Prevention, 2023), accessed December 6, 2024, https://www.cdc.gov/breastfeeding-data/media /pdfs/2024/06/2022-Breastfeeding-Report-Card-508.pdf.

Chapter 1: What to Expect from Bottle Service

7 *at their baby's half birthday*: *Breastfeeding Report Card: United States, 2022* (Centers for Disease Control and Prevention, 2023), accessed December 6, 2024, https://www.cdc.gov/breastfeeding-data/media /pdfs/2024/06/2022-Breastfeeding-Report-Card-508.pdf.

7 *Willow, Bobbie, and SimpliFed*: The State of Feeding, accessed December 6, 2024, https://stateoffeeding.com/.

8 *instructed by a health care provider*: "Chapter 3: Infant Feeding," Centers for Disease Control and Prevention, July 1, 2024, accessed December 19, 2024, https://www.cdc.gov/breastfeeding-data/media /pdfs/2024/05/ifps2_tables_ch3.pdf.

8 *how long they would breastfeed*: *2023 Infant Feeding Survey: Key Findings* (Infant Nutrition Council of America, 2023), accessed March 2, 2025, https://infantnutrition.org/wp-content/uploads /2024/04/Key-Findings-2023-Infant-Feeding-Survey.pdf.

8 *feeling proud about using formula*: The State of Feeding, 2024.

8 *reported feeling judged*: "Mothers and Caregivers Need Comprehensive Information on Feeding Infants," GQR Insights and Action,

accessed December 9, 2024, https://infantnutrition.org/wp-content
/uploads/2024/04/Infant-Feeding-Survey.pdf.

8   *In a 2021 Wakefield study*: *The 2021 Feeding Confessionals Report*
(Bobbie x Wakefield Research, 2021), accessed March 2, 2025,
https://cdn2.hubspot.net/hubfs/20958570/The_2021_Feeding
_Confessionals_Report.pdf.

11   *bulk of feeding duties*: Lizzie Aviv et al., *The Fair Play Method: Can
We Solve for the Unequal Division of Domestic Labor?* (Fair Play
Policy Institute, 2024), accessed March 2, 2025, https://publicex
change.usc.edu/wp-content/uploads/2024/11/PX_FairPlay-Final
-Report_Dec2024.pdf.

Chapter 2: What Is Baby Formula?

13   *there has never been a time*: Emily E. Stevens et al., "A History of Infant Feeding," *Journal of Perinatal Education* 18, no. 2 (Spring 2009):
32–39, https://doi.org/10.1624/105812409X426314.

14   *was first noted*: Ian G. Wicks, "A History of Infant Feeding: Part 1.
Primitive Peoples: Ancient Works: Renaissance Writers," *Archives of
Disease in Childhood* 28, no. 138 (April 1953): 151–58, https://doi
.org/10.1136/adc.28.138.151.

14   *primary method of alternative feeding*: M. L. Osborn, "The Rent
Breasts: A Brief History of Wet-Nursing," *Midwife, Health Visitor &
Community Nurse* 15, no. 8 (1979): 302–6, https://pubmed.ncbi
.nlm.nih.gov/381849/.

14   *"a feasible substitute"*: Stevens et al., "A History of Infant Feeding."

14   *from as early as 2000 BCE*: Wicks, "A History of Infant Feeding."

14   *used for infant feeding*: Fred Weinberg, "Infant Feeding Through the
Ages," *Canadian Family Physician* 39 (September 1993): 2016–20,
https://pmc.ncbi.nlm.nih.gov/articles/instance/2379896/pdf
/canfamphys00115-0164.pdf.

14   *"pap" or "panada"*: Samuel X. Radbill, "Infant Feeding Through the
Ages," *Clinical Pediatrics* 20, no. 10 (1981): 613–21, https://doi.org
/10.1177/000992288102001001.

14 *formula was developed*: Radbill, "Infant Feeding."

14 *different brands of infant foods*: Samuel J. Fomon, "Infant Feeding in the 20th Century: Formula and Beikost," *Journal of Nutrition* 131 (2001): 409S–20S, https://doi.org/10.1093/jn/131.2.409S.

14 *Committee on Foods was formed*: Stevens et al., "A History of Infant Feeding."

15 *"inspection requirements"*: Raymond E. Newberry, "The Infant Formula Act of 1980," *Journal of Association of Official Analytical Chemists* 65, no. 6 (1982): 1472–73, https://doi.org/10.1093/jaoac/65.6.1472.

15 FDA regulatory requirements: "Infant Formula," FDA, December 2, 2024, accessed December 12, 2024, https://www.fda.gov/food/resources-you-food/infant-formula.

15 *most highly regulated foods*: Wayne F. Wargo, "The History of Infant Formula: Quality, Safety, and Standard Methods," *Journal of AOAC International* 99, no. 1 (2016): 7–11, https://doi.org/10.5740/jaoacint.15-0244.

16 *critical developmental period*: Sian Robinson, "Infant Nutrition and Lifelong Health: Current Perspectives and Future Challenges," *Journal of Developmental Origins of Health and Disease* 6, no. 5 (2015): 384–89, https://doi.org/10.1017/S2040174415001257.

16 *what is found in breast milk*: Daniel J. Raiten et al., "LSRO Report: Assessment of Nutrient Requirements for Infant Formulas," *Journal of Nutrition* 128, no. 11 (1998): 2059S–293S, https://doi.org/10.1093/jn/128.suppl_11.2059S.

16 *an effective substitute*: Camila R. Martin et al., "Review of Infant Feeding: Key Features of Breast Milk and Infant Formula," *Nutrients* 8, no. 5 (2016): 279, https://doi.org/10.3390/nu8050279.

16 *hormones, antibodies, stem cells, and growth factors*: Olivia Ballard and Ardythe L. Morrow, "Human Milk Composition: Nutrients and Bioactive Factors," *Pediatric Clinics of North America* 60, no. 1 (2013): 49–74, https://doi.org/10.1016/j.pcl.2012.10.002.

16 *very similar to breast milk*: Martin et al., "Review of Infant Feeding."

16 *harmful substances called* antigens: "Medical Dictionary of Health Terms: A–C," Harvard Health Publishing, December 13, 2011, accessed December 16, 2024, https://www.health.harvard.edu/a-through-c.

17 *only last a few weeks or months*: "Immunity Types," Centers for Disease Control and Prevention, July 30, 2024, accessed December 19, 2024, https://www.cdc.gov/vaccines/basics/immunity-types.html.

17 *pacifier use and group childcare*: Bernard Branger et al., "Breastfeeding and Respiratory, Ear and Gastro-Intestinal Infections, in Children, Under the Age of One Year, Admitted Through the Paediatric Emergency Departments of Five Hospitals," *Frontiers in Pediatrics* 10 (February 2023): 1–12, https://doi.org/10.3389/fped.2022.1053473.

18 *do well on this type of formula*: Dina M. DiMaggio et al., "Updates in Infant Nutrition," *Pediatrics in Review* 38, no. 10 (2017): 449–62, https://doi.org/10.1542/pir.2016-0239.

18 *crying, fussiness, colic symptoms, and gas*: Ronald E. Kleinman and Frank R. Greer, *Pediatric Nutrition*, 8th ed. (American Academy of Pediatrics, 2020), 89–98.

18 harder *to digest, not easier*: Arissara Phosanam et al., "In Vitro Digestion of Infant Formula Model Systems: Influence of Casein to Whey Protein Ratio," *International Dairy Journal* 117 (February 2021): 105008, https://doi.org/10.1016/j.idairyj.2021.105008.

19 *will not react*: Committee on Nutrition, "Hypoallergenic Infant Formulas," *Pediatrics* 106, no. 2 (2000): 346–49, https://doi.org/10.1542/peds.106.2.346.

20 *less popular than powder formula*: Victor Oliveira et al., "WIC and the Retail Price of Infant Formula," *Food Assistance and Nutrition Research Report*, no. 39 (May 2004): 26, https://www.ers.usda.gov/webdocs/publications/46787/15976_fanrr39-1_1_.pdf.

21 *Powdered formula is not sterile*: "Infant Formula Preparation and Storage," Centers for Disease Control and Prevention, May 16, 2023, accessed December 16, 2024, https://www.cdc.gov/nutrition/InfantandToddlerNutrition/formula-feeding/infant-formula-preparation-and-storage.html.

Chapter 3: Bottle Feeding from Birth–Planning Ahead

25 *Emily Oster's book* Cribsheet: Emily Oster, *Cribsheet: A Data-Driven Guide to Better, More Relaxed Parenting, from Birth to Preschool* (Penguin, 2020).

30 *feeding at the breast*: Dee Kassing, "Bottle-Feeding as a Tool to Reinforce Breastfeeding," *International Lactation Consultant Association* 18, no. 1 (2002), https://doi.org/10.1177/089033440201800110.

Chapter 4: Drying Up Your Milk (Whenever You're Ready)

31 *stage two lactogenesis*: "Lactation," Cleveland Clinic, December 16, 2021, accessed February 28, 2025, https://my.clevelandclinic.org/health/body/22201-lactation.

32 *medication(s) to suppress lactation*: Olufemi T. Oladapo and Bukola Fawole, "Treatments for Suppression of Lactation," *Cochrane Database of Systematic Reviews*, no. 9 (September 2012): CD005937, https://doi.org/10.1002/14651858.CD005937.pub3.

32 *used for this purpose in 1994*: "Bromocriptine," Drugs and Lactation Database (LactMed®), National Institute of Child Health and Human Development, September 15, 2024, accessed February 28, 2025, https://www.ncbi.nlm.nih.gov/books/NBK501306/.

32 *sued the FDA*: "F.D.A. Is Sued on Drug to Dry Mothers' Milk," *New York Times*, August 17, 1994, accessed February 28, 2025, https://www.nytimes.com/1994/08/17/us/fda-is-sued-on-drug-to-dry-mothers-milk.html.

32 *between 1980 and 1994*: David R. Olmos, "Sandoz to Stop Selling Parlodel as Treatment to Halt Lactation: Pharmaceuticals: Company Defends the Drug, Calls the Move 'a Business Decision' in the Face of Consumer Pressure," *Los Angeles Times*, August 19, 1994, accessed February 28, 2025, https://www.latimes.com/archives/la-xpm-1994-08-19-fi-29031-story.html.

33 *altogether too quickly*: "Drying Up Your Breasts (Weaning)," Children's Healthcare of Atlanta, 2023, accessed February 28, 2025,

https://www.choa.org/-/media/Files/Childrens/teaching-sheets
/rapid-weaning---drying-up-your-breasts.pdf.

33   *no longer encouraged*: Kathy Swift, "Breast Binding . . . Is It All That
It's Wrapped Up to Be?" *Journal of Obstetric, Gynecologic & Neonatal Nursing* 32, no. 3 (2003): 332–39, https://doi.org/10.1177
/0884217503253531.

34   *in some research studies*: I. Zakarija-Grkovic and F. Stewart, "Treatments for Breast Engorgement During Lactation (Review),"
Cochrane Database of Systematic Reviews, no 9. (2020): CD006946,
https://doi.org/10.1002%2F14651858.CD006946.pub4.

34   *to provide relief*: Kathryn L. Roberts et al., "Effects of Cabbage Leaf
Extract on Breast Engorgement," *Journal of Human Lactation* 14, no.
3 (1998): 231–36, https://doi.org/10.1177/089033449801400312.

34   *Drink sage tea*: Anne Eglash, "Treatment of Maternal Hypergalactia,"
Breastfeeding Medicine 9, no. 9 (2014): 423–25, https://doi.org
/10.1089/bfm.2014.0133.

34   *Peppermint oil*: Eglash, "Treatment of Maternal Hypergalactia."

35   *suppression of milk production*: "Peppermint," Drugs and Lactation
Database (LactMed®), National Institute of Child Health and Human Development, January 15, 2025, accessed February 28, 2025,
https://www.ncbi.nlm.nih.gov/books/NBK501851/.

35   *should be diluted*: "How to Dilute Peppermint Oil?" Nikura, September 23, 2023, accessed February 28, 2025, https://nikura.com/blogs
/essential-oils/how-to-dilute-peppermint-oil.

35   *Apply ice packs*: "Drying Up Your Breasts (Weaning)," Children's
Healthcare of Atlanta, 2023, accessed February 28, 2025, https://
www.choa.org/-/media/Files/Childrens/teaching-sheets/rapid
-weaning---drying-up-your-breasts.pdf.

35   *reduce milk supply in lactating women*: Helen M. Johnson et al.,
"ABM Clinical Protocol #32: Management of Hyperlactation,"
Breastfeeding Medicine 15, no. 3 (2020): 129–34, https://doi.org
/10.1089/bfm.2019.29141.hmj.

35 *nearly 25 percent reduction*: Khalidah Aljazaf et al., "Pseudoephedrine: Effects on Milk Production in Women and Estimation of Infant
   Exposure via Breastmilk," *British Journal of Clinical Pharmacology*
   56, no. 1 (2003): 18–24, https://doi.org/10.1046/j.1365
   2125.2003.01822.x.

35 *increased blood pressure and heart rate*: Stephen M. Salerno et al.,
   "Effect of Oral Pseudoephedrine on Blood Pressure and Heart Rate:
   A Meta-Analysis," *Archives of Internal Medicine* 165, no. 15 (2005):
   1686–94, https://doi.org/10.1001/archinte.165.15.1686.

35 *nausea, and headaches*: "Pseudoephedrine," MedlinePlus, February
   15, 2018, accessed February 28, 2025, https://medlineplus.gov
   /druginfo/meds/a682619.html.

36 *developing mastitis*: "Mastitis and Sore Breasts," La Leche League
   International, July 2023, accessed February 28, 2025, https://llli.org
   /breastfeeding-info/mastitis/.

Chapter 5: Choosing a Baby Formula

41 *to meet the nutrient levels*: Raymond E. Newberry, "The Infant
   Formula Act of 1980," *Journal of Association of Official Analytical
   Chemists* 65, no. 6 (1982): 1472–73, https://doi.org/10.1093/jaoac
   /65.6.1472.

41 *at a similar level*: "21 CFR 107.100," Food and Drug Administration
   Department of Health and Human Services, accessed December 19,
   2024, https://www.ecfr.gov/current/title-21/part-107/section
   -107.100.

43 *"routine" or "standard" formula*: Dina M. DiMaggio et al., "Updates
   in Infant Nutrition," *Pediatrics in Review* 38, no. 10 (2017): 449–62,
   https://doi.org/10.1542/pir.2016-0239.

43 *are considered safe*: Yvan Vandenplas et al., "Partially Hydrolyzed Formula in Non-Exclusively Breastfed Infants: A Systematic Review and
   Expert Consensus," *Nutrition* 57 (May 2018): 0899-9007, https://
   doi.org/10.1016/j.nut.2018.05.018.

43 *40 percent casein protein*: Clemens Kunz and Bo Lonnerdal, "Re-
    evaluation of the Whey Protein/Casein Ratio of Human Milk,"
    Acta Paediatrica 81, no. 2 (1992): 107–12, https://doi.org/10.1111
    /j.1651-2227.1992.tb12184.x.

43 *a type of beta-casein protein*: Michele J. Sadler and Nicholas Smith,
    "Beta-Casein Proteins and Infant Growth and Development," *Infant
    Journal* 9, no. 5 (2013): 173–76, https://www.infantjournal.co.uk
    /pdf/inf_053_tei.pdf.

43 *20 percent whey protein*: Sadler and Smith, "Beta-Casein Proteins."

44 *calories that come from breast milk*: Su Yeong Kim and Dae Yong
    Yi, "Components of Human Breast Milk: From Macronutrient to
    Microbiome and MicroRNA," *Clinical and Experimental Pediatrics*
    63, no. 8 (2020): 301–9, https://doi.org/10.3345/cep.2020.00059/.

44 *source in breast milk is lactose*: Olivia Ballard and Ardythe L. Mor-
    row, "Human Milk Composition: Nutrients and Bioactive Factors,"
    Pediatric Clinics of North America 60, no. 1 (2013): 49–74, https://
    doi.org/10.1016/j.pcl.2012.10.002.

44 *lactating parent consumes dairy*: Daphna K. Dror and Lindsay H.
    Allen, "Overview of Nutrients in Human Milk," *Advances in Nutri-
    tion* 9, no. 1 (2018): 278S–94S, https://doi.org/10.1093/advances
    /nmy022.

44 *begin producing lactase*: Munir Mobassaleh et al., "Development of
    Carbohydrate Absorption in the Fetus and Neonate," *Pediatrics* 75,
    no. 1 (1985): 160–66, https://doi.org/10.1542/peds.75.1.160.

45 *congenital lactase deficiency*: Melvin B. Heyman, "Lactose Intolerance
    in Infants, Children, and Adolescents," *Pediatrics* 118, no. 3 (2006):
    1279–86, https://doi.org/10.1542/peds.2006-1721.

45 *goat's milk fat*: Sophie Gallier et al., "Whole Goat Milk as a Source of
    Fat and Milk Fat Globule Membrane in Infant Formula," *Nutrients*
    12, no. 11 (2020): 3486, https://www.mdpi.com/2072-6643/12/11
    /3486.

46 *an infant could suffer*: Shilpa N. Bhupathiraju and Frank Hu, "Es-
    sential Fatty Acid Deficiency," Merck Manual Professional Version,

October 2023, accessed January 16, 2025, https://www.merckmanu als.com/professional/nutritional-disorders/undernutrition/essential -fatty-acid-deficiency.

47 *sold in the US must contain*: "21 CFR 107.100," Food and Drug Administration.

47 *throughout the first year*: "Where We Stand: Vitamin D & Iron Supplements for Babies," American Academy of Pediatrics, May 24, 2022, accessed January 16, 2025, https://www.healthychildren.org /English/ages-stages/baby/feeding-nutrition/Pages/Vitamin-Iron -Supplements.aspx.

47 *1.8 mg of iron per 100-calorie serving*: Alexander Strzalkowski et al., "Iron and DHA in Infant Formula Purchased in the US Fails to Meet European Nutrition Requirements," *Nutrients* 15, no. 8 (2023): 1812, https://doi.org/10.3390/nu15081812.

47 *higher-than-average risk*: "Anemia in Children and Teens: Parent FAQs," American Academy of Pediatrics, January 24, 2019, accessed January 16, 2025, https://www.healthychildren.org/English/health -issues/conditions/chronic/Pages/Anemia-and-Your-Child.aspx.

48 *when added to infant formula*: Cristine Couto Almeida et al., "Bioactive Compounds in Infant Formula and Their Effects on Infant Nutrition and Health: A Systematic Literature Review," *International Journal of Food Science*, May 2021, https://onlinelibrary.wiley.com /doi/10.1155/2021/8850080.

Chapter 6: Getting Over the Guilt

57 *fed formula at some point*: *Breastfeeding Report Card: United States, 2022* (Centers for Disease Control and Prevention, 2023), accessed February 28, 2025, https://www.cdc.gov/breastfeeding-data/media /pdfs/2024/06/2022-Breastfeeding-Report-Card-508.pdf.

60 *thirty-two ounces of formula per day*: "Vitamin D for Babies, Children & Adolescents," American Academy of Pediatrics, August 24, 2022, accessed January 16, 2025, https://www.healthychildren.org /English/healthy-living/nutrition/Pages/vitamin-d-on-the-double.aspx.

Chapter 7: How to Make a Bottle (and How to Make Your Life Easier)

63 how to make a bottle of formula: "Chapter 3. Infant Feeding," Centers for Disease Control and Prevention, July 1, 2024, accessed December 19, 2024, https://www.cdc.gov/breastfeeding-data/media /pdfs/2024/05/ifps2_tables_ch3.pdf.

63 *baby turns six months old*: *Breastfeeding Report Card: United States, 2022* (Centers for Disease Control and Prevention, 2023), accessed December 6, 2024, https://www.cdc.gov/breastfeeding-data/media /pdfs/2024/06/2022-Breastfeeding-Report-Card-508.pdf.

64 Wash your hands: "Handling Infant Formula Safely: What You Need to Know," Food and Drug Administration, May 17, 2024, accessed January 16, 2025, https://www.fda.gov/food/buy-store-serve-safe -food/handling-infant-formula-safely-what-you-need-know.

64 *more susceptible to infections*: Laszlo Marodi, "Neonatal Innate Immunity to Infectious Agents," *Infection and Immunity* 74, no. 4 (2006): 1999–2006, https://journals.asm.org/doi/10.1128/iai.74.4.1999 -2006.2006.

64 *(no need for antibacterial soap)*: "Hand Washing: A Powerful Antidote to Illness," American Academy of Pediatrics, February 7, 2022, accessed January 16, 2025, https://www.healthychildren.org/English /health-issues/conditions/prevention/Pages/Hand-Washing-A -Powerful-Antidote-to-Illness.aspx.

66 *Tap water*: "Infant Formula Preparation and Storage," Centers for Disease Control and Prevention, December 19, 2024, accessed January 16, 2025, https://www.cdc.gov/infant-toddler-nutrition /formula-feeding/preparation-and-storage.html.

66 *Distilled water; purified water*: "Infants, Formula, and Fluoride," *Journal of the American Dental Association* 138, no. 1 (2007): 132, https://jada.ada.org/article/S0002-8177(14)61101-6/fulltext.

66 *not recommended for daily formula consumption include: Tap water*: "Infant Formula Preparation and Storage," CDC.

66 *Well water*: Alan Woolf, "Is Your Drinking Water Safe?," American Academy of Pediatrics, February 22, 2023, accessed January 16, 2025, https://www.healthychildren.org/English/safety-prevention /all-around/Pages/Is-Your-Drinking-Water-Safe.aspx.

67 *boiling the water*: Steven A. Abrams, "How to Safely Prepare Baby Formula with Water," American Academy of Pediatrics, January 4, 2024, accessed January 16, 2025, https://www.healthychildren.org /English/ages-stages/baby/formula-feeding/Pages/how-to-safely -prepare-formula-with-water.aspx.

67 *The FDA recommends this for infants*: "Handling Infant Formula Safely," FDA.

67 does *need to be diluted with water*: "Handling Infant Formula Safely," FDA.

67 *punch-type can opener is recommended*: "Bottle Feeding Formula Preparation," Nationwide Children's Hospital, 2021, accessed January 23, 2025, https://www.nationwidechildrens.org/family -resources-education/health-wellness-and-safety-resources/helping -hands/bottle-feeding-formula-preparation.

67 *a one-to-one ratio*: "Handling Infant Formula Safely," FDA.

69 *(but not in the refrigerator)*: "Handling Infant Formula Safely," FDA.

69 *within twenty-four hours if serving later*: "Infant Formula Preparation and Storage," CDC.

70 *remember 24:2:1*: "Infant Formula Preparation and Storage," CDC.

70 *likelihood that bacteria*: "How to Prepare and Store Powdered Formula (CDC)," NeoKit, June 16, 2023, accessed January 23, 2025, https://publications.aap.org/neokit/white-paper-parent/23728 /How-to-Prepare-and-Store-Powdered-Formula-CDC.

73 *lead to gas and discomfort*: "Gas Relief for Babies," American Acade-my of Pediatrics, January 7, 2025, accessed January 23, 2025, https:// www.healthychildren.org/English/ages-stages/baby/diapers-clothing /Pages/Breaking-Up-Gas.aspx.

Chapter 8: Position Matters (When It Comes to Feeding)

78 *position the baby more like this*: Dee Kassing, "Bottle-Feeding as a Tool to Reinforce Breastfeeding," *Journal of Human Lactation* 18, no. 1 (2002): 56–60, https://www.bfar.org/bottlefeeding.pdf.

80 *breathing, sucking, and swallowing*: Kassing, "Bottle-Feeding as a Tool."

80 *rates more similar to breastfeeding*: Alison K. Ventura et al., "Does Paced Bottle-Feeding Improve the Quality and Outcome of Bottle-Feeding Interactions," *Early Human Development* 201 (February 2025): 106181, https://doi.org/10.1016/j.earlhumdev.2024.106181.

80 *may make a big difference*: "How to Help a Newborn with Gas," Children's Hospital of Philadelphia, September 26, 2024, accessed January 27, 2025, https://www.chop.edu/news/health-tip/how-help-newborn-gas.

81 *tightness in the neck muscles*: Henri Aarnivala et al., "Preventing Deformational Plagiocephaly through Parent Guidance: A Randomized, Controlled Trial," *European Journal of Pediatrics* 174, no. 9 (2015): 1197–208, https://doi.org/10.1007/s00431-015-2520-x.

81 *positional plagiocephaly*: Tristain de Chalain et al., "Torticollis Associated with Positional Plagiocephaly: A Growing Epidemic," *Journal of Craniofacial Surgery* 16, no. 3 (May 2005): 411–18, https://doi.org/10.1097/01.scs.0000171967.47358.47.

81 *sleep deprivation*: Baian A. Baattaiah et al., "The Relationship between Fatigue, Sleep Quality, Resilience, and the Risk of Postpartum Depression: An Emphasis on Maternal Mental Health," *BMC Psychology* 11, no. 1 (2023): 1–17, https://doi.org/10.1186/s40359-023-01043-3.

Chapter 9: What's Normal, What's Not, and When to Switch Formulas

86 *immature digestive systems*: Hanyun Jiang et al., "Development of the Digestive System in Early Infancy and Nutritional Management of

Digestive Problems in Breastfed and Formula-Fed Infants," *Food & Function* 13, no. 3 (2022): 1062–77, https://doi.org/10.1039 /d1fo03223b.

86 *develops over time*: Flavia Indrio et al., "Development of the Gastrointestinal Tract in Newborns as a Challenge for an Appropriate Nutrition: A Narrative Review," *Nutrients* 14, no. 7 (2022): 1405, https:// doi.org/10.3390/nu14071405.

86 *This is a ring of muscle*: Ryan D. Rosen and Ryan Winters, "Physiology, Lower Esophageal Sphincter," StatPearls, March 17, 2023, accessed February 6, 2025, https://www.ncbi.nlm.nih.gov/books /NBK557452/.

87 *we tend to see reflux*: Cincinnati Children's Health Library, "Gastroesophageal Reflux in Infants," June 2023, accessed February 6, 2025, https://www.cincinnatichildrens.org/health/g/ger-infants.

87 *second and third trimesters of pregnancy*: I. Antonowicz and E. Lebenthal, "Developmental Pattern of Small Intestinal Enterokinase and Disaccharidase Activities in The Human Fetus," *Gastroenterology* 72, no. 6 (1977): 1299–303, https://pubmed.ncbi.nlm.nih.gov /558125/.

87 *sufficient lactase enzymes*: Melvin B. Heyman, "Lactose Intolerance in Infants, Children, and Adolescents," *Pediatrics* 118, no. 3 (2006): 1279–86, https://doi.org/10.1542/peds.2006-1721.

87 *gut microbiota compared to other age groups*: Yao Yao et al., "The Role of Microbiota in Infant Health: From Early Life to Adulthood," *Frontiers in Immunology* 12 (October 2021), https://doi.org /10.3389/fimmu.2021.708472.

88 *health and overall nutrition are influenced*: Giulia Catassi et al., "The Role of Diet and Nutritional Interventions for the Infant Gut Microbiome," *Nutrients* 16, no. 3 (2024): 400, https://doi.org /10.3390/nu16030400.

88 *may take in too much air*: Eugene C. Goldfield et al., "Coordination of Sucking, Swallowing, and Breathing and Oxygen Saturation During Early Infant Breast-Feeding and Bottle-Feeding," *Pediatric*

Research 60 (2006): 450–55, https://www.nature.com/articles
/pr2006270.

88 *which can make them uncomfortable*: Mashette Syrkin-Nikolau and
Hannibal Person, "Abdominal Pain in Infants: 8 Possible Reasons
Your Baby's Tummy Hurts," American Academy of Pediatrics, May 8,
2023, accessed February 6, 2025, https://www.healthychildren.org
/English/health-issues/conditions/abdominal/Pages/Abdominal
-Pains-in-Infants.aspx.

88 *gas can also cause reflux*: "Reflux in Babies," Cleveland Clinic, March
4, 2024, accessed February 5, 2025, https://my.clevelandclinic.org
/health/diseases/reflux-in-babies.

89 *around twelve weeks*: Syrkin-Nikolau and Person, "Abdominal Pain
in Infants."

89 *resolve over the course of the first year*: Marlene Curien-Chotard
and Prevost Jantchou, "Natural History of Gastroesophageal Reflux
in Infancy: New Data from A Prospective Cohort," *BMC Pediatrics*
20, no. 152 (2020), https://bmcpediatr.biomedcentral.com/articles
/10.1186/s12887-020-02047-3.

89 *volume and positioning*: Anthony Porto, "Gastroesophageal Reflux
(GER) & Gastroesophageal Reflux Disease (GERD)," American
Academy of Pediatrics, December 29, 2024, accessed February 7,
2025, https://www.healthychildren.org/English/health-issues
/conditions/abdominal/Pages/GERD-Reflux.aspx.

89 *some babies are starting to roll*: Courtney J. Wusthoff, "Movement
Milestones: Birth to 3-Months," American Academy of Pediatrics,
August 12, 2020, accessed February 7, 2025, https://www.healthy
children.org/English/ages-stages/baby/Pages/Movement-Birth-to
-Three-Months.aspx.

89 *may trigger increased reflux*: "Reflux (Spitting Up)," Seattle Children's, February 2, 2025, accessed February 7, 2025, https://www
.seattlechildrens.org/conditions/a-z/reflux-spitting-up/.

90 *every few days*: Emilie Moretti et al., "The Bowel Movement Characteristics of Exclusively Breastfed and Exclusively Formula Fed Infants

Differ During the First Three Months of Life," *Acta Paediatrica* 108, no. 5 (May 2019): 877–81, https://doi.org/10.1111/apa.14620.

90 *even if they have bowel movements infrequently*: Barton Schmitt, "Constipation," American Academy of Pediatrics, 2024, accessed February 7, 2025, https://www.healthychildren.org /English/tips-tools/symptom-checker/Pages/symptomviewer .aspx?symptom=Constipation.

90 *can be an indication of an allergy*: Alexandra K. Martinson, "Cow's Milk Protein Allergy," First 1000 Day's Knowledge Center, February 2024, accessed February 8, 2025, https://publications.aap.org /first1000days/module/28106/Cow-s-Milk-Protein-Allergy.

91 *comes in small amounts*: Barton Schmitt, "Spitting Up—Reflux," American Academy of Pediatrics, 2024, accessed February 8, 2025, https://www.healthychildren.org/English/tips-tools/symptom-check er/Pages/symptomviewer.aspx?symptom=Spitting+Up+-+Reflux.

91 *should always be evaluated*: Barton Schmitt, "Rash or Redness— Widespread," American Academy of Pediatrics, 2024, accessed February 8, 2025, https://www.healthychildren.org /English/tips-tools/symptom-checker/Pages/symptomviewer .aspx?symptom=Rash+or+Redness+-+Widespread.

91 *indication of an allergy*: Rita Nocerino et al., "The Controversial Role of Food Allergy in Infantile Colic: Evidence and Clinical Management," *Nutrients* 7, no. 3 (2015): 2015–25, https://doi.org/10.3390 /nu7032015.

93 *Five S's framework*: Happiest Baby Staff, "The Science of the 5 S's," Happiest Baby, accessed January 23, 2025, https://www.happiest baby.com/blogs/baby/science-5-s-s.

95 *a form of torture*: Hilary Andersson, "Stop! I Can't Stand It!" BBC Sounds, accessed January 25, 2025, https://www.bbc.co.uk/sounds /play/p0356m6q.

95 *gets better by three months*: Dieter Wolke et al., "Crying Durations and Prevalence of Colic in Infants," *Journal of Pediatrics* 185 (June 2017): 55–61, https://doi.org/10.1016/j.jpeds.2017.02.020.

96 *impact on new moms' mental health*: Michaela Nagl et al., "Social
Media Use and Postpartum Body Image Dissatisfaction: The Role of
Appearance-Related Social Comparisons and Thin-Ideal Internaliza-
tions," *Midwifery* 100 (September 2021): 103038, https://doi.org
/10.1016/j.midw.2021.103038.

99 *keep your attention*: Christophe Haubursin, "It's Not You. Phones are
Designed to Be Addicting," *Vox*, February 27, 2018, accessed January
27, 2025, https://www.vox.com/2018/2/27/17053758/phone
-addictive-design-google-apple.

101 *lower well-being*: James A. Roberts and Meredith E. David, "On the
Outside Looking In: Social Media Intensity, Social Connection, and
User Well-Being: The Moderating Role of Passive Social Media Use,"
Canadian Journal of Behavioural Science 55, no. 3 (2023): 240–42,
https://doi.org/10.1037/cbs0000323.

Chapter 10: Why Is Pooping So Hard?

104 infant dyschezia: Cathrine Gatzinsky, "Bowel Habits in Healthy
Infants and the Prevalence of Functional Constipation, Infant Colic
and Infant Dyschezia," *Acta Paediatrica* 112, no. 6 (2023): 1341–50,
https://doi.org/10.1111/apa.16736.

104 *coordinate the muscles*: "Patient & Family Education Materials: Infant
Dyschezia," Children's Minnesota, 2025, accessed February 9, 2025,
https://www.childrensmn.org/educationmaterials/childrensmn
/article/21819/infant-dyschezia/.

104 *first weeks or months after birth*: "Patient & Family Education,"
Children's Minnesota.

105 *green, yellow, or brown*: Laura Jana and Jennifer Shu, "The Many
Colors of Baby Poop," American Academy of Pediatrics, July 11,
2024, accessed February 9, 2025, https://www.healthychildren.org
/English/ages-stages/baby/Pages/The-Many-Colors-of-Poop.aspx.

105 *iron that formula is fortified with*: J. S. Hyams, "Effect of Infant Formula on Stool Characteristics of Young Infants," *Pediatrics* 95, no. 1
(1995): 50–54, https://pubmed.ncbi.nlm.nih.gov/7770309/.

105 *evaluated by your child's doctor*: Jana and Shu, "The Many Colors of Baby Poop."

105 *The most common, normal textures*: N. L. H. Bekkali, "Constipation in Infancy and Childhood: New Insights into Pathophysiological Aspects and Treatment," University of Amsterdam, 2010, accessed February 9, 2025, https://pure.uva.nl/ws/files/1294622/73258_07.pdf.

105 *infant's stool texture*: Bekkali, "Constipation in Infancy and Childhood."

105 *palm olein oil*: John B. Lasekan et al., "Impact of Palm Olein in Infant Formulas on Stool Consistency and Frequency: A Meta-Analysis of Randomized Clinical Trials," *Food & Nutrition Research* 61, no. 1 (2017): 1330104, https://doi.org/10.1080 /16546628.2017.1330104.

106 *contribute to firmer stools*: Edgardo. E. Malacaman et al., "Effect of Protein Source and Iron Content of Infant Formula on Stool Characteristics," *Journal of Pediatric Gastroenterology and Nutrition* 4, no. 5 (1985): 771–73, https://doi.org/10.1002/j.1536-4801.1985 .tb08953.x.

106 *Parents may notice looser stools*: Shang-Ling Wu et al., "Growth, Gastrointestinal Tolerance and Stool Characteristics of Healthy Term Infants Fed an Infant Formula Containing Hydrolyzed Whey Protein (63%) and Intact Casein (37%): A Randomized Clinical Trial," *Nutrients* 9, no. 11 (2017): 1254, https://doi.org/10.3390 /nu9111254.

106 *should follow up on*: "Baby Poop Guide," Children's Hospital Colorado, October 19, 2020, accessed February 10, 2025, https://www .childrenscolorado.org/just-ask-childrens/articles/baby-poop-guide/.

106 *challenge with lactose*: Pamela Sylvia Douglas, "Diagnosing Gastro-Oesophageal Reflux Disease or Lactose Intolerance in Babies Who Cry a Lot in the First Few Months Overlooks Feeding Problems," *Journal of Paediatrics and Child Health* 49, no. 4 (2013): E252–56, https://doi.org/10.1111/jpc.12153.

106 *These may include*: Barton Schmitt, "Constipation," American Academy of Pediatrics, 2024, accessed February 10, 2025, https://

www.healthychildren.org/English/tips-tools/symptom-checker/Pages/symptomviewer.aspx?symptom=Constipation.

106 *poop five times a day*: Emilie Moretti et al., "The Bowel Movement Characteristics of Exclusively Breastfed and Exclusively Formula Fed Infants Differ During the First Three Months of Life," *Acta Paediatrica* 108, no. 5 (2019): 877–81, https://doi.org/10.1111/apa.14620.

107 *Infrequency is typically only a problem*: "Rome IV Criteria: Appendix A: Rome IV Diagnostic Criteria for FGIDs," Rome Foundation, accessed February 10, 2025, https://theromefoundation.org/rome-iv/rome-iv-criteria/.

107 *even if it doesn't happen often*: "Constipation in Infants and Children," National Library of Medicine Medline Plus, July 31, 2024, accessed February 10, 2025, https://medlineplus.gov/ency/article/003125.htm.

107 *every-other-day routine*: Schmitt, "Constipation."

107 *identifiable pieces of food*: "12 Types of Baby Poop & What They Mean," UnityPoint Health, accessed February 10, 2025, https://www.unitypoint.org/news-and-articles/12-types-of-baby-poop-what-they-mean-infographic.

108 *a sign of something underlying*: Rachel Nall, "Why Is There Mucus in My Baby's Poop?" Healthline, February 14, 2023, accessed February 10, 2025, https://www.healthline.com/health/mucus-in-baby-poop.

108 secondary lactase deficiency: Talia F. Malik and Kiran K. Panuganti, "Lactose Intolerance," StatPearls, April 17, 2023, accessed February 10, 2025, https://www.ncbi.nlm.nih.gov/books/NBK532285/.

108 *produce lactase enzymes*: Melvin B. Heyman, "Lactose Intolerance in Infants, Children, and Adolescents," *Pediatrics* 118, no. 3 (2006): 1,279–86, https://doi.org/10.1542/peds.2006-1721.

109 *continuing breast milk in all cases*: Heyman, "Lactose Intolerance."

109 *younger than three months or malnourished*: Heyman, "Lactose Intolerance."

109 *beyond what's consumed via breast milk or infant formula*: Natalie
D. Muth, "Recommended Drinks for Children Age 5 & Younger,"
American Academy of Pediatrics, October 3, 2023, accessed February 10, 2025, https://www.healthychildren.org/English/healthy
-living/nutrition/Pages/recommended-drinks-for-young-children
-ages-0-5.aspx.

109 *softer, easier stools*: M. M. Tabbers et al., "Evaluation and Treatment
of Functional Constipation in Infants and Children: Evidence-Based
Recommendations from ESPGHAN and NASPGHAN," *Journal of
Pediatric Gastroenterology and Nutrition* 58, no. 2 (2014): 258–74,
https://doi.org/10.1097/MPG.0000000000000266.

109 *preventing diaper rash*: Barton Schmitt, "Diaper Rash," American
Academy of Pediatrics, 2024, accessed February 10, 2025, https://
www.healthychildren.org/English/tips-tools/symptom-checker
/Pages/symptomviewer.aspx?symptom=Diaper+Rash.

110 *hands can give you a clue*: "Signs Your Child Is Hungry or Full," CDC
Infant and Toddler Nutrition, October 21, 2024, accessed December
11, 2024, https://www.cdc.gov/infant-toddler-nutrition/mealtime
/signs-your-child-is-hungry-or-full.html.

Chapter 11: The Inconsistency of Nipple Flows

118 *nipples across brands*: Britt Frisk Pados et al., "Milk Flow Rates from
Bottle Nipples Used After Hospital Discharge," *MCN: The American Journal of Maternal/Child Nursing* 41, no. 4 (2016): 237–43,
https://doi.org/10.1097/NMC.0000000000000244.

118 *gagging, increased drooling, and coughing*: "Choosing a Bottle Flow
Rate," Nationwide Children's Hospital, accessed February 10, 2025,
https://www.nationwidechildrens.org/family-resources-education
/health-wellness-and-safety-resources/helping-hands/choosing-a
-bottle-flow-rate.

118 *Too fast a flow*: Mashette Syrkin-Nikolau and Hannibal Person,
"Abdominal Pain in Infants: 8 Possible Reasons Your Baby's Tummy
Hurts," American Academy of Pediatrics, May 8, 2023, accessed
February 10, 2025, https://www.healthychildren.org/English

/health-issues/conditions/abdominal/Pages/Abdominal-Pains-in
-Infants.aspx.

118 *depending on the brand*: Pados et al., "Milk Flow Rates."

119 *Nipple Flow Rate Is Too Fast*: "Choosing a Bottle Flow Rate," Nationwide Children's Hospital.

120 *Nipple Flow Rate Is Too Slow*: "Choosing a Bottle Flow Rate,"
Nationwide Children's Hospital.

121 *for up to twenty-four hours*: "Handling Infant Formula Safely: What
You Need to Know," Food and Drug Administration, May 17, 2024,
accessed January 16, 2025, https://www.fda.gov/food/buy-store
-serve-safe-food/handling-infant-formula-safely-what-you-need-know.

123 *mixing had time to break up*: Zafir Gaygadzhiev, "Investigating the
Impact of Processing Conditions on the Emulsion Stability, Viscos-
ity, and Foaming Capacity of Concentrated Infant Formula Emul-
sions," *Applied Food Research* 3, no. 1 (2023): 100294, https://doi
.org/10.1016/j.afres.2023.100294.

Chapter 12: Supplementing and Combo Feeding

132 *Common reasons for combo feeding*: Carmen Monge-Montero et al.,
"Why Do Mothers Mix Milk Feed Their Infants? Results from a
Systematic Review," *Nutrition Reviews* 82, no. 10 (2024): 1355–71,
https://doi.org/10.1093/nutrit/nuad134.

135 *a supply and demand model*: Steven E. J. Daly et al., "Infant Demand
and Milk Supply. Part 1: Infant Demand and Milk Production in
Lactating Women," *Journal of Human Lactation* 11, no. 1 (1995):
21–26, https://doi.org/10.1177/089033449501100119.

135 *robust milk supply*: "Low Milk Supply," WIC Breastfeeding Support,
US Department of Agriculture, accessed February 28, 2025, https://
wicbreastfeeding.fns.usda.gov/low-milk-supply.

136 *a formula feeding a day*: "Introducing Formula Feeds," National Health
Service (UK), accessed February 28, 2025, https://www.nhs.uk
/start-for-life/baby/feeding-your-baby/mixed-feeding/introducing
-formula-feeds/.

136 *stool color (yellow to green)*: Laura Jana and Jennifer Shu, "The Many Colors of Baby Poop," American Academy of Pediatrics, July 11, 2024, accessed February 28, 2025, https://www.healthy children.org/English/ages-stages/baby/Pages/The-Many-Colors -of-Poop.aspx.

136 *frequency (more to less)*: Laura A. Jana and Jennifer Shu, "Pooping by the Numbers: What's Normal for Infants?" American Academy of Pediatrics, July 11, 2024, accessed February 28, 2025, https://www .healthychildren.org/English/ages-stages/baby/Pages/Pooping-By -the-Numbers.aspx.

Chapter 13: Getting Ready for Day Care, a Nanny, or a Trustworthy Friend

137 *spending five minutes underwater*: TODAY Parents (@todayparents), "I quit my job to stay home . . ," Facebook, July 27, 2020, https:// www.facebook.com/todayparents/photos/i-quit-my-job-to-stay -home-when-i-had-my-second-baby-just-after-her-big-brother -/10157795706277984/.

138 *twenty-four hours in the refrigerator*: "Handling Infant Formula Safely: What You Need to Know," Food and Drug Administration, May 17, 2024, accessed January 16, 2025, https://www.fda.gov/food /buy-store-serve-safe-food/handling-infant-formula-safely-what-you -need-know.

140 *to be used for another feeding*: "Handling Infant Formula Safely," FDA.

145 *Signs and symptoms of postpartum anxiety*: "Postpartum Anxiety," Cleveland Clinic, April 12, 2022, accessed February 18, 2025, https://my.clevelandclinic.org/health/diseases/22693-postpartum -anxiety.

146 *take off twelve to eighteen months*: "US Department of Labor An-nounces New Research that Underscores Benefits of Paid Family and Medical Leave," United States Department of Labor, November 21, 2024, accessed February 27, 2025, https://www.dol.gov/newsroom /releases/wb/wb20241121.

146 *Canada*: "EI maternity and parental benefits," Government of Canada, February 4, 2025, accessed February 27, 2025, https://www.canada.ca/en/services/benefits/ei/ei-maternity-parental.html.

146 *the UK*: "Maternity Pay and Leave," Government Digital Service, Part of Department for Science, Innovation and Technology, UK, accessed February 27, 2025, https://www.gov.uk/maternity-pay-leave/pay.

146 *Australia*: "How Much You Can Get," Australian Government—Services Australia, December 9, 2024, accessed February 27, 2025, https://www.servicesaustralia.gov.au/how-much-parental-leave-pay-you-can-get-for-child-born-or-adopted-from-1-july-2023?context=64479.

146 *"We may not always be there"*: Laura Hunter and Jennifer Walker, *Moms on Call: Basic Baby Care 0–6 Months* (Moms on Call, 2006).

148 *healthy attachment is influenced*: National Collaborating Centre for Mental Health (UK), "Introduction to Children's Attachment" in *Children's Attachment: Attachment in Children and Young People Who Are Adopted from Care, in Care or at High Risk of Going into Care* (National Institute for Health and Care Excellence, 2015), https://www.ncbi.nlm.nih.gov/books/NBK356196/.

148 *also influence attachment*: Nazmi Mutlu Karakas and Figen Sahin Dagli, "The Importance of Attachment in Infant and Influencing Factors," *Turkish Archives of Pediatrics* 54, no. 2 (2019): 76–81, https://doi.org/10.14744/TurkPediatriArs.2018.80269.

149 *parents did in generations past*: "Parents Now Spend Twice as Much Time with Their Children as 50 Years Ago," *Economist*, November 27, 2017, accessed February 18, 2025, https://www.economist.com/graphic-detail/2017/11/27/parents-now-spend-twice-as-much-time-with-their-children-as-50-years-ago.

Chapter 14: Traveling with Formula

152 *sucking is known to help soothe*: Laura A. Jana and Jennifer Shu, "Practical Pacifier Principles," American Academy of Pediatrics, November 19, 2009, accessed February 28, 2025, https://www.healthychildren

.org/English/ages-stages/baby/crying-colic/Pages/Practical-Pacifier
-Principles.aspx.

154 *provides guidance*: "Baby Formula," Transportation Security Administration, US Department of Homeland Security, accessed February
28, 2025, https://www.tsa.gov/travel/security-screening/whatcan
ibring/items/baby-formula.

157 *tubes that connect the middle ear*: Yamini Durani, "Flying and Your
Child's Ears," Nemours KidsHealth, September 2023, accessed February 28, 2025, https://kidshealth.org/en/parents/flying-ears.html.

160 *into your arms for each bottle feeding*: Michelle Pratt, "Can You Feed
a Baby in a Car Seat," Safe in the Seat, January 24, 2025, accessed
February 28, 2025, https://www.safeintheseat.com/post/can-you
-feed-a-baby-in-a-car-seat.

160 *increase risk of ear infections*: "Ear Infections," *Paediatrics Child
Health* 14, no. 7 (2009): 465–66, https://doi.org/10.1093/pch
/14.7.465.

160 *in the case of a crash*: Pratt, "Can You Feed a Baby."

Chapter 15: Introducing a Schedule

162 *feed your baby on demand*: "Is Your Baby Hungry or Full? Responsive
Feeding Explained," American Academy of Pediatrics, August 13,
2024, accessed February 20, 2024, https://www.healthychildren.org
/English/ages-stages/baby/feeding-nutrition/Pages/Is-Your-Baby
-Hungry-or-Full-Responsive-Feeding-Explained.aspx.

163 *longer stretches of sleep at night*: Christophe Mühlematter et al.,
"Not Simply a Matter of Parents—Infants' Sleep-Wake Patterns Are
Associated with Their Regularity of Eating," *PLOS One* 18, no. 10
(2023): e0291441, https://doi.org/10.1371/journal.pone.0291441.

164 *missing calories at night*: Amy Brown and Victoria Harries, "Infant
Sleep and Night Feeding Patterns During Later Infancy: Association with Breastfeeding Frequency, Daytime Complementary Food
Intake, and Infant Weight," *Breastfeeding Medicine* 10, no. 5 (2015),
https://doi.org/10.1089/bfm.2014.0153.

164 *in the early months*: Sanjeev Jain and Maya Bunik, "How Often and How Much Should Your Baby Eat?," American Academy of Pediatrics, April 2, 2024, accessed February 20, 2025, https://www.healthychildren.org/English/ages-stages/baby/feeding-nutrition/Pages/how-often-and-how-much-should-your-baby-eat.aspx.

164 *consistent wake time every morning*: "Sleep in Infants (2–12 Months)," Nationwide Children's, accessed February 20, 2025, https://www.nationwidechildrens.org/specialties/sleep-disorder-center/sleep-in-infants.

166 *come from formula or breast milk*: "Starting Solid Foods," American Academy of Pediatrics, August 12, 2022, accessed February 20, 2025, https://www.healthychildren.org/English/ages-stages/baby/feeding-nutrition/Pages/Starting-Solid-Foods.aspx.

166 *thirty-two ounces of breast milk or formula*: "Amount and Schedule of Baby Formula Feedings," American Academy of Pediatrics, May 16, 2022, accessed February 20, 2025, https://www.healthychildren.org/English/ages-stages/baby/formula-feeding/Pages/amount-and-schedule-of-formula-feedings.aspx.

166 *Check with your pediatrician*: Jain and Bunik, "How Often and How Much."

169 *feeding that takes place*: Gwen Dewar, "Dream Feeding: An Evidence-Based Guide to Helping Babies Sleep Longer," Parenting Science, July 2022, accessed February 20, 2025, https://parentingscience.com/dream-feeding/.

170 *helps your baby sleep longer*: Mirja Quante et al., "Associations of Sleep-Related Behaviors and the Sleep Environment at Infant Age One Month with Sleep Patterns in Infants Five Months Later," *Sleep Medicine* 91 (June 2022): 31–37, https://doi.org/10.1016/j.sleep.2022.03.019.

171 *to sleep through the night*: "Infant Sleep," Children's Hospital of Philadelphia, accessed February 20, 2025, https://www.chop.edu/primary-care/infant-sleep.

171 *regular sleep schedules*: "Sleep," American Academy of Pediatrics, accessed February 20, 2025, https://www.healthychildren.org /English/ages-stages/baby/sleep/Pages/default.aspx.

171 *upright for some time*: Barton Schmitt, "Spitting Up—Reflux," American Academy of Pediatrics, 2024, accessed February 20, 2025, https://www.healthychildren.org/English/tips-tools/symptom -checker/Pages/symptomviewer.aspx?symptom=Spitting+Up+ -+Reflux.

Chapter 16: To Feed or Not to Feed? Dealing with Night Wakings

174 *wake at night to eat*: "Sleep in Your Baby's First Year," Cleveland Clinic, June 15, 2023, accessed February 24, 2025, https:// my.clevelandclinic.org/health/articles/14300-sleep-in-your -babys-first-year.

174 *exhibit the following signs*: "Signs Your Child Is Hungry or Full," CDC Infant and Toddler Nutrition, October 21, 2024, accessed February 24, 2025, https://www.cdc.gov/infant-toddler-nutrition /mealtime/signs-your-child-is-hungry-or-full.html.

175 *jerk their arms and legs* in their sleep: Anastasis Georgoulas et al., "Sleep–Wake Regulation in Preterm and Term Infants," *Sleep* 44, no. 1 (2020): zsaa148, https://doi.org/10.1093/sleep/zsaa148.

175 *observe before intervening*: Rachel Moon, "Sleeping Like a Baby: Stories & Tips From the Front Lines," American Academy of Pediat-rics, September 11, 2023, accessed February 24, 2025, https://www .healthychildren.org/English/healthy-living/sleep/Pages/sleeping -like-a-baby-restless-nights-and-tips-from-the-front-lines.aspx.

176 *occurs only in breastfed babies*: Karen Gill, "How to Break the Pattern of Reverse Cycling," Healthline, March 24, 2016, accessed February 24, 2025, https://www.healthline.com/health/parenting /reverse-cycling.

178 *about half an hour less*: Mirja Quante et al., "Associations of Sleep-Related Behaviors and the Sleep Environment at Infant Age One Month with Sleep Patterns in Infants Five Months Later,"

Sleep Medicine 91 (June 2022): 31–37, https://doi.org/10.1016
/j.sleep.2022.03.019.

178 *two to five minutes before taking action*: Craig Canapari, "How to Use
the 'Le Pause' Method to Help Your Baby Sleep Better," June 5, 2024,
accessed February 20, 2025, https://drcraigcanapari.com/le-pause
-avoiding-sleep-problems-and-why-you-wont-break-your-kids/.

179 *can soothe*: Harvey Karp, "The 5 S's for Soothing Babies," Happiest
Baby, accessed February 20, 2025, https://www.happiestbaby.com
/blogs/baby/the-5-s-s-for-soothing-babies#3.-shushing.

179 *"nipple confusion"*: E. Zimmerman, "Clarifying Nipple Confusion,"
Journal of Perinatology 35 (July 2015): 895–99, https://doi.org
/10.1038/jp.2015.83.

179 *reduces the likelihood of SIDS*: Fern R. Hauck et al., "Do Pacifiers
Reduce the Risk of Sudden Infant Death Syndrome? A Meta-
Analysis," *Pediatrics* 116, no. 5 (2005): e716–23, https://doi.org
/10.1542/peds.2004-2631.

179 *calm an agitated baby*: Karp, "The 5 S's."

Chapter 17: You're Not Crazy: There Is More Spit-Up

182 *reflux peaks*: "Reflux in Babies," Cleveland Clinic, March 4, 2024,
accessed February 20, 2025, https://my.clevelandclinic.org/health
/diseases/reflux-in-babies.

182 *the contents of the stomach*: Jenifer R. Lightdale et al., "Gastroesophageal Reflux: Management Guidance for the Pediatrician," *Pediatrics*
131, no. 5 (2013): e1684–95, https://publications.aap.org
/pediatrics/article/131/5/e1684/31266/Gastroesophageal-Reflux
-Management-Guidance-for.

183 *reduce by the three-month mark*: Mashette Syrkin-Nikolau and Han-
nibal Person, "Abdominal Pain in Infants: 8 Possible Reasons Your
Baby's Tummy Hurts," American Academy of Pediatrics, May 8,
2023, accessed February 7, 2025, https://www.healthychildren.org
/English/health-issues/conditions/abdominal/Pages/Abdominal
-Pains-in-Infants.aspx.

183 *reflux tends to get worse*: Syrkin-Nikolau and Person, "Abdominal Pain in Infants."

183 *more spit-up between three and six months of age*: Alejandro Velez and Christine Waasdorp Hurtado, "Why Babies Spit Up," American Academy of Pediatrics, January 3, 2025, accessed February 24, 2025, https://www.healthychildren.org/English/ages-stages/baby/feeding -nutrition/Pages/Why-Babies-Spit-Up.aspx.

183 *again at six months*: "Cluster Feeding and Growth Spurts," WIC Breastfeeding Support, accessed February 24, 2025, https://wic breastfeeding.fns.usda.gov/cluster-feeding-and-growth-spurts.

184 *nearer to the six-month mark*: "Infant Food and Feeding," American Academy of Pediatrics, November 28, 2023, accessed February 24, 2025, https://www.aap.org/en/patient-care/healthy-active-living -for-families/infant-food-and-feeding.

184 *if your child has reflux*: Anthony Porto, "Gastroesophageal Reflux (GER) & Gastroesophageal Reflux Disease (GERD)," American Academy of Pediatrics, December 29, 2024, accessed February 24, 2025, https://www.healthychildren.org/English/health-issues /conditions/abdominal/Pages/GERD-Reflux.aspx.

184 *Symptoms of GERD can include*: Rachel Rosen et al., "Pediatric Gastroesophageal Reflux Clinical Practice Guidelines: Joint Recommendations of the North American Society for Pediatric Gastroenterology, Hepatology, and Nutrition (NASPGHAN) and the European Society for Pediatric Gastroenterology, Hepatology, and Nutrition (ESPGHAN)," *Journal of Pediatric Gastroenterology and Nutrition* 66, no. 3 (2018): 516–54, https://doi.org/10.1097 /MPG.0000000000001889.

186 *reflux will resolve over time*: Barton Schmitt, "Spitting Up—Reflux," American Academy of Pediatrics, 2024, accessed February 24, 2025, https://www.healthychildren.org/English/tips-tools/symptom -checker/Pages/symptomviewer.aspx?symptom=Spitting+Up+ -+Reflux.

186 *bottle is relatively level*: Schmitt, "Spitting Up—Reflux."

186 *Avoid Overfeeding*: Velez and Hurtado, "Why Babies Spit Up."

186 *Get Out a Good Burp*: Velez and Hurtado, "Why Babies Spit Up."

187 *this isn't the only way to get them to burp*: "Baby Burping, Hiccups & Spit-Up," American Academy of Pediatrics, December 31, 2024, accessed February 24, 2025, https://www.healthychildren.org /English/ages-stages/baby/feeding-nutrition/Pages/baby-burping -hiccups-and-spit-up.aspx.

187 *Keep 'Em Upright*: Schmitt, "Spitting Up—Reflux."

187 *liquids to leave the stomach*: Neha S. Kwatra, "Gastric Emptying of Milk in Infants and Children Up to 5 Years of Age: Normative Data and Influencing Factors," *Pediatric Radiology* 50, no. 5 (2020): e689–97, https://doi.org/10.1007/s00247-020-04614-3.

188 *Ensure Correct Nipple Flow*: Schmitt, "Spitting Up—Reflux."

189 *some research exists to support their benefit*: Jann P. Foster, "Probiotics for Preventing and Treating Infant Regurgitation: A Systematic Review and Meta-Analysis," *Maternal & Child Nutrition* 18, no. 1 (2021): e13290, https://pmc.ncbi.nlm.nih.gov/articles /PMC8710121/.

189 *adequate evidence to support its use*: Laura A. Jana and Jennifer Shu, "Gas Relief for Babies," American Academy of Pediatrics, January 7, 2025, accessed February 24, 2025, https://www.healthychildren.org /English/ages-stages/baby/diapers-clothing/Pages/Breaking-Up-Gas .aspx.

189 *Try a Hypoallergenic Formula*: Rosen et al., "Pediatric Gastroesophageal Reflux."

189 *Other Oral Motor Issues*: Mark H. Fishbein et al., "A Multidisciplinary Approach to Infants With GERD-Like Symptoms: A New Paradigm," *Journal of Pediatric Gastroenterology and Nutrition* 77, no. 1 (2023): 39–46, https://doi.org/10.1097 /MPG.0000000000003802.

190 *dysfunction in the muscles in the mouth*: "What Is a Speech-Language Pathologist," Cleveland Clinic, January 12, 2023, accessed February 24, 2025, https://my.clevelandclinic.org/health/articles /24602-speech-language-pathologist.

190 *no longer recommended for sleep*: "About Feeding from a Bottle," CDC Infant and Toddler Nutrition, March 25, 2024, accessed February 24, 2025, https://www.cdc.gov/infant-toddler-nutrition /bottle-feeding/index.html.

190 *experience gastroesophageal reflux*: Rosen et al., "Pediatric Gastro-esophageal Reflux."

190 *safe source for thickening*: "Oatmeal: The Safer Alternative for Infants & Children Who Need Thicker Food," American Academy of Pediatrics, April 18, 2016, accessed February 24, 2025, https://www .healthychildren.org/English/health-issues/conditions/abdominal /Pages/Oatmeal-The-Safer-Alternative-Need-Thicker-Food.aspx.

190 *after forty-two weeks gestational age*: Rosen et al., "Pediatric Gastro-esophageal Reflux."

190 *Talk to your child's pediatrician about thickeners*: Laura A. Jana and Jennifer Shu, "Cereal in a Bottle: Solid Food Shortcuts to Avoid," American Academy of Pediatrics, May 14, 2015, accessed February 24, 2025, https://www.healthychildren.org/English/ages-stages /baby/feeding-nutrition/Pages/Cereal-in-a-Bottle-Solid-Food -Shortcuts-to-Avoid.aspx.

191 *Try Reflux Medication*: Rosen et al., "Pediatric Gastroesophageal Reflux."

191 *improve with age*: Schmitt, "Spitting Up—Reflux."

Chapter 18: Milk Stays King! Balancing Food and Formula

202 *healthy eating pattern*: *Dietary Guidelines for Americans*, 9th ed., (US Department of Agriculture and US Department of Health and Human Services, 2020–2025), https://www.dietaryguidelines.gov /sites/default/files/2020-12/Dietary_Guidelines_for_Americans _2020-2025.pdf.

203 *Solids are important for*: *Dietary Guidelines for Americans*.

203 *different flavors, textures*: I. Blossfeld et al., "Texture Preferences of 12-Month-Old Infants and the Role of Early Experiences," *Food*

Quality and Preference 18, no. 2 (2007): 396–404, https://doi.org /10.1016/j.foodqual.2006.03.022.

203   *mouth and jaw*: Hermann Kalhoff et al., "Development of Eating Skills in Infants and Toddlers from a Neuropediatric Perspective," *Italian Journal of Pediatrics* 50, no. 110 (2024), https://doi.org /10.1186/s13052-024-01683-0.

203   *mealtimes with their caregivers*: Charlotte Webber et al., "An Infant-Led Approach to Complementary Feeding Is Positively Associated with Language Development," *Maternal & Child Nutrition* 17, no. 4 (2021): e13206, https://doi.org/10.1111/mcn.13206.

204   *engage in responsive feeding*: Ronald E. Kleinman and Frank R. Greer, *Pediatric Nutrition*, 8th ed. (American Academy of Pediatrics, 2020), 163–86.

204   *eat the foods that you offer*: Ellyn Satter, "Ellyn Satter's Division of Responsibility in Feeding," 2015, accessed February 25, 2025, https://www.ellynsatterinstitute.org/wp-content/uploads/2015/08 /ELLYN-SATTER%E2%80%99S-DIVISION-OF-RESPONSIBIL ITY-IN-FEEDING.pdf.

205   *new flavors and textures become acceptable*: "Infant Food and Feeding," American Academy of Pediatrics, November 28, 2023, accessed February 25, 2025, https://www.aap.org/en/patient-care/healthy -active-living-for-families/infant-food-and-feeding/.

205   *a greater amount of healthy fats*: Kleinman and Greer, *Pediatric Nutrition*.

207   *second half of their first year*: *Dietary Guidelines for Americans*.

208   *exposure to arsenic found in rice*: "Oatmeal: The Safer Alternative for Infants & Children Who Need Thicker Food," American Academy of Pediatrics, April 18, 2016, accessed February 27, 2025, https:// www.healthychildren.org/English/health-issues/conditions/abdomi nal/Pages/Oatmeal-The-Safer-Alternative-Need-Thicker-Food.aspx.

208   *should not be frozen*: "Handling Infant Formula Safely: What You Need to Know," Food and Drug Administration, May 17, 2024,

accessed February 24, 2025, https://www.fda.gov/food/buy-store
-serve-safe-food/handling-infant-formula-safely-what-you-need-know.

209 *reduce the risk of food allergies*: David M. Fleischer et al., "A Consensus
Approach to the Primary Prevention of Food Allergy Through Nutri-
tion: Guidance from the American Academy of Allergy, Asthma, and
Immunology; American College of Allergy, Asthma, and Immunol-
ogy; and the Canadian Society for Allergy and Clinical Immunol-
ogy," *Journal of Allergy and Clinical Immunology: In Practice* 9, no. 1
(2021): 22–43, https://www.aaaai.org/Aaaai/media/Media-Library
-PDFs/Allergist%20Resources/Statements%20and%20Practice%20
Parameters/A-Consensus-Approach-to-the-Primary-Prevention-of
-Food-Allergy-Through-Nutrition-Jan-21-(1).pdf.

211 *at least twelve years of age*: "Car Seats and Booster Seats," National
Highway Traffic Safety Administration, US Department of Transportation, accessed February 25, 2025, https://www.nhtsa.gov
/vehicle-safety/car-seats-and-booster-seats.

211 *expressly discouraged now*: "About Feeding from a Bottle," CDC Infant and Toddler Nutrition, March 25, 2024, accessed February 24,
2025, https://www.cdc.gov/infant-toddler-nutrition/bottle-feeding
/index.html.

211 *around six months*: "Starting Solid Foods," American Academy of
Pediatrics, August 12, 2022, accessed February 25, 2025, https://
www.healthychildren.org/English/ages-stages/baby/feeding
-nutrition/Pages/Starting-Solid-Foods.aspx.

211 *can no longer be sold*: "New Federal Crib Rules Go into Effect
Tomorrow," Department of Consumer Protection, June 27, 2011,
accessed February 25, 2025, https://portal.ct.gov/dcp/news-releases
-from-the-department-of-consumer-protection/2011-news-releases
/new-federal-crib-rules-go-into-effect-tomorrow?language=en_US.

Chapter 19: There Are a Million Right Ways to Start Solids

216 *go-to method for starting solids in infancy*: Amy Bentley,
Inventing Baby Food: Taste, Health, and the Industrialization

of the American Diet (University of California Press, 2014), accessed February 25, 2025, https://doi.org/10.1525/california /9780520277373.003.0005.

216   *starting with rice cereal*: Karen Gill, "When Is It Safe to Feed Your Baby Rice Cereal?" Healthline, April 9, 2020, accessed February 25, 2025, https://www.healthline.com/health/baby/when-can-you -start-feeding-a-baby-rice-cereal.

216   *advised to move to*: Darlene Martin, "Introducing Solid Foods to Baby," Historical Materials from University of Nebraska–Lincoln Extension, 1990, accessed February 25, 2025, https://digitalcommons .unl.edu/extensionhist/801.

216   *prefer to start with them*: Amy Brown and Michelle Lee, "A Descriptive Study Investigating the Use and Nature of Baby-Led Weaning in a UK Sample of Mothers," *Maternal & Child Nutrition* 7, no. 1 (2010), https://doi.org/10.1111/j.1740-8709.2010.00243.x.

217   *Current guidance from the AAP*: Ronald E. Kleinman and Frank R. Greer, *Pediatric Nutrition*, 8th ed. (American Academy of Pediatrics, 2020), 163–86.

217   *introducing the next food*: "When, What, and How to Introduce Solid Foods," CDC Infant and Toddler Nutrition, December 5, 2023, accessed February 27, 2025, https://www.cdc.gov/infant -toddler-nutrition/foods-and-drinks/when-what-and-how-to -introduce-solid-foods.html.

217   *this practice may not be necessary*: David M. Fleischer et al., "A Consensus Approach to the Primary Prevention of Food Allergy Through Nutrition: Guidance from the American Academy of Allergy, Asthma, and Immunology; American College of Allergy, Asthma, and Immunology; and the Canadian Society for Allergy and Clinical Immunology," *Journal of Allergy and Clinical Immunology: In Practice* 9, no. 1 (2021): 22–43, https://www.aaaai.org/Aaaai/media/Media -Library-PDFs/Allergist%20Resources/Statements%20and%20Prac tice%20Parameters/A-Consensus-Approach-to-the-Primary -Prevention-of-Food-Allergy-Through-Nutrition-Jan-21-(1).pdf.

217   *consistent exposure is important*: Fleischer et al., "A Consensus Approach."

218   *eat throughout toddlerhood*: W. Stewart Agras et al., "Improving Healthy Eating in Families with a Toddler at Risk for Overweight: A Cluster Randomized Controlled Trial," *Journal of Developmental & Behavioral Pediatrics* 33, no. 7 (2012): 529–34, https://doi.org /10.1097/DBP.0b013e3182618e1f.

218   *steak is best served*: Rachel Ruiz et al., "Steak," Solid Starts, accessed February 25, 2025, https://solidstarts.com/foods/steak.

218   *Solid Starts*: Solid Starts, accessed February 25, 2025, https://solid starts.com/.

218   *100 foods before 1*: Katie Ferraro, "100 Foods for Your Baby to Try Before Turning One," 2017, accessed February 25, 2025, https:// calwic.org/wp-content/uploads/2019/06/Katie-Ferraro_100Foods _hmv2.pdf.

218   *wide variety of foods*: Meera D. Patel et al., "Considering Nature and Nurture in the Etiology and Prevention of Picky Eating: A Narrative Review," *Nutrients* 12, no. 11 (2020): 3409, https://doi.org/10.3390 /nu12113409.

220   *due to risk of botulism*: "Botulism," American Academy of Pediatrics, November 19, 2018, accessed February 25, 2025, https://www .healthychildren.org/English/health-issues/conditions/infections /Pages/Botulism.aspx.

220   *pasteurized and raw honey*: "Botulism," World Health Organization, September 25, 2023, accessed February 25, 2025, https://www.who .int/news-room/fact-sheets/detail/botulism.

220   *added sugar and/or high in salt*: "Foods and Drinks to Avoid or Lim- it," CDC Infant and Toddler Nutrition, December 4, 2023, accessed February 25, 2025, https://www.cdc.gov/infant-toddler-nutrition /foods-and-drinks/foods-and-drinks-to-avoid-or-limit.html.

220   *water and formula or breast milk*: "Foods and Drinks to Avoid."

220   *High-mercury fish*: "Foods and Drinks to Avoid."

220   *contain less mercury*: "Advice About Eating Fish," US Food and
      Drug Administration and United States Environmental Protection
      Agency, October 2021, accessed February 25, 2025, https://www
      .fda.gov/media/102331/download.

220   *Choking hazards*: "Choking Hazards," CDC Infant and Toddler
      Nutrition, October 10, 2024, accessed February 25, 2025, https://
      www.cdc.gov/infant-toddler-nutrition/foods-and-drinks/choking
      -hazards.html.

221   *By preparing foods safely*: "Reducing the Risk of Choking in Young
      Children at Mealtimes," United States Department of Agriculture
      Food and Nutrition Service, September 2020, accessed February 25,
      2025, https://wicworks.fns.usda.gov/sites/default/files/media
      /document/English_ReducingRiskofChokinginYoungChildren.pdf.

224   *foods like avocado*: "Sample Menu for a Baby 8 to 12 Months Old,"
      American Academy of Pediatrics, August 12, 2022, accessed Febru-
      ary 26, 2025, https://www.healthychildren.org/English/ages-stages
      /baby/feeding-nutrition/Pages/sample-one-day-menu-for-an-8-to
      -12-month-old.aspx.

225   *fruits and vegetables at age six*: Kirsten A. Grimm et al., "Fruit and
      Vegetable Intake During Infancy and Early Childhood," *Pediatrics*
      134, no. 1 (2014): S63-S69, https://doi.org/10.1542/peds.2014
      -0646K.

226   *before a baby might try it*: Patel et al., "Considering Nature and
      Nurture."

227   *will eventually accept them*: Patel et al., "Considering Nature and
      Nurture."

Chapter 20: Cups, Up! Introducing a Cup

229   *solids at around six months old*: Jennifer Shu, "From Bottle to Cup:
      Helping Your Child Make a Healthy Transition," American Academy
      of Pediatrics, July 3, 2023, accessed February 27, 2025, https://www
      .healthychildren.org/English/ages-stages/baby/feeding-nutrition
      /Pages/Discontinuing-the-Bottle.aspx.

229 *a small open cup*: Megan McNamee, "Teach Your Baby or Toddler How to Drink from a Variety of Cups," Feeding Littles, accessed February 27, 2025, https://feedinglittles.com/blogs/blog/the-ultimate-guide-to-cup-drinking.

230 *this hasn't been proven*: Stefanie LaManna, "Skip the Sippy? Coaching Parents on Sippy Cup Use," ASHA (American Speech-Language-Hearing Association) LeaderLive, October 24, 2024, accessed February 27, 2025, https://leader.pubs.asha.org/do/10.1044/2024-1023-sippy-cups-slps/full/.

230 *a straw cup is another good option*: Melanie Potock, "Sippy Cups: 3 Reasons to Skip Them and What to Offer Instead," ASHA (American Speech-Language-Hearing Association) LeaderLive, February 28, 2017, accessed February 27, 2025, https://leader.pubs.asha.org/do/10.1044/sippy-cups-3-reasons-to-skip-them-and-what-to-offer-instead/full/.

231 *hard-spouted sippy cups*: LaManna, "Skip the Sippy?"

231 *recommended to be introduced*: LaManna, "Skip the Sippy?"

232 *small amounts of water*: *Dietary Guidelines for Americans*, 9th ed. (US Department of Agriculture and US Department of Health and Human Services, 2020–2025), https://www.dietaryguidelines.gov/sites/default/files/2020-12/Dietary_Guidelines_for_Americans_2020-2025.pdf.

232 *toddlers under twelve months of age*: *Dietary Guidelines for Americans*.

232 *Keep bottles and cups focused on*: *Dietary Guidelines for Americans*.

232 *in small amounts*: *Dietary Guidelines for Americans*.

232 *AAP's recommendation*: Shu, "From Bottle to Cup."

233 *descend and position themselves*: Shu, "From Bottle to Cup."

233 *starting at around six months of age*: *Dietary Guidelines for Americans*.

234 *encouraged to transition to a cup*: Shu, "From Bottle to Cup."

Chapter 21: How to Drop a Bottle

240 *four to five bottle feedings per day*: "Amount and Schedule of Baby Formula Feedings," American Academy of Pediatrics, May 16, 2022, accessed February 26, 2025, https://www.healthychildren.org /English/ages-stages/baby/formula-feeding/Pages/amount-and -schedule-of-formula-feedings.aspx.

240 *eight ounces . . . in each*: Natalie D. Muth, "Recommended Drinks for Children Age 5 & Younger," American Academy of Pediatrics, October 3, 2023, accessed February 26, 2025, https://www.healthy children.org/English/healthy-living/nutrition/Pages/Recommended -Drinks-for-Young-Children-Ages-0-5.aspx.

241 *per pound of body weight*: "Amount and Schedule of Baby Formula Feedings."

241 *remove between four and twelve months*: "Amount and Schedule of Baby Formula Feedings."

242 *any remaining night feedings*: Barton Schmitt, "Bottle-Feeding (Formula) Questions," American Academy of Pediatrics, 2024, accessed February 26, 2025, https://www.healthychildren.org /English/tips-tools/symptom-checker/Pages/symptomviewer .aspx?symptom=Bottle-Feeding+(Formula)+Questions.

243 *twelve through twenty-four months*: Muth, "Recommended Drinks."

248 *per pound of body weight than infants*: Unaiza Faizan and Audra S. Rouster, "Nutrition and Hydration Requirements in Children and Adults," StatPearls, August 28, 2023, accessed February 26, 2025, https://www.ncbi.nlm.nih.gov/books/NBK562207/.

248 *the rate of growth slows down*: Morey Haymond et al., "Early Recognition of Growth Abnormalities Permitting Early Intervention," *Acta Paediatrica* 102, no. 8 (2013): 787–96, https://doi.org/10.1111/apa.12266.

Chapter 22: Trading Formula for Milk

253 *toddlers ages one to two*: Natalie D. Muth, "Recommended Drinks for Children Age 5 & Younger," American Academy of Pediatrics,

October 3, 2023, accessed February 26, 2025, https://www.healthy children.org/English/healthy-living/nutrition/Pages/Recommended -Drinks-for-Young-Children-Ages-0-5.aspx.

254 *One cup of whole milk contains*: US Department of Agriculture, "Milk, Whole, 3.25% Milkfat, with Added Vitamin D," FoodData Central Food Details, December 16, 2019, accessed February 28, 2025, https://fdc.nal.usda.gov/food-details/746782/nutrients.

254 *similar nutrition to cow's milk*: Sokratis Stergiadis et al., "Comparative Nutrient Profiling of Retail Goat and Cow Milk," *Nutrients* 11, no. 10 (2019): 2282, https://doi.org/10.3390/nu11102282.

254 *compared to A1 beta-casein proteins*: Sae-In S. Kay, "Beneficial Effects of Milk Having A2 β-Casein Protein: Myth or Reality?" *Journal of Nutrition* 151, no. 5 (2021): 1061–72, https://doi.org/10.1093/jn /nxaa454.

254 *cow's milk protein allergy*: Olga Benjamin-van Aalst, "Goat Milk Allergy and a Potential Role for Goat Milk in Cow's Milk Allergy," *Nutrients* 16, no. 15 (2024): 2402, https://doi.org /10.3390/nu16152402.

255 *protein, vitamin D, and calcium*: Muth, "Recommended Drinks."

255 *Pea milk*: Muth, "Recommended Drinks."

255 *Oat milk*: Muth, "Recommended Drinks."

256 *does not recommend toddler formulas*: Muth, "Recommended Drinks."

256 *not nutritionally equivalent, or even close, to whole cow's milk*: Muth, "Recommended Drinks."

257 *talk to your pediatrician*: Claire McCarthy, "My Preschooler Refuses to Drink Milk. What Should We Do?" American Academy of Pediatrics, November 18, 2016, accessed February 28, 2025, https:// www.healthychildren.org/English/tips-tools/ask-the-pediatrician /Pages/My-preschooler-refuses-to-drink-milk.aspx.

257 *combining milk in the same bottle*: "Making the Switch to Cow's Milk for 1-Year-Olds," Children's Hospital of Philadelphia, September 27,

2024, accessed February 28, 2025, https://www.chop.edu/news /making-switch-cow-s-milk-1-year-olds.

259 *twenty-four ounces per day*: Anthony Porto and Rachel Drake, "Cow's Milk Alternatives: Parent FAQs," HealthyChildren.org, June 2, 2022, accessed February 28, 2025, https://www.healthychildren.org /English/healthy-living/nutrition/Pages/milk-allergy-foods-and -ingredients-to-avoid.aspx.

259 *too much milk per day can result*: Karolina Graczykowska, "The Consequence of Excessive Consumption of Cow's Milk: Protein-Losing Enteropathy with Anasarca in the Course of Iron Deficiency Anemia—Case Reports and a Literature Review," *Nutrients* 13, no. 3 (2021): 828, https://doi.org/10.3390/nu13030828.

260 *Managing Constipation Post-Milk Introduction*: Barton Schmitt, "Constipation," American Academy of Pediatrics, 2024, accessed February 28, 2025, https://www.healthychildren.org /English/tips-tools/symptom-checker/Pages/symptomviewer .aspx?symptom=Constipation.

Chapter 23: Quitting the Bottle Altogether

266 *when to discontinue bottle use*: Morium B. Bably et al., "Age of Bottle Cessation and BMI-for-Age Percentile Among Children Aged Thirty-Six Months Participating in WIC," *Childhood Obesity* 18, no. 3 (2022), 197–205, https://doi.org/10.1089/chi.2021.0119.

266 *require different muscle coordination to use*: Dorota Cudzilo, "Infant and Baby Feeding and the Development of the Maxillofacial Complex Based on Own Observations and the Literature," *Developmental Period Medicine* 22, no. 3 (2018): 255–59, https://doi.org/10.34763 /devperiodmed.20182203.255259.

266 *speech development in toddlerhood*: Jennifer Shu, "From Bottle to Cup: Helping Your Child Make a Healthy Transition," American Academy of Pediatrics, July 3, 2023, accessed February 27, 2025, https://www.healthychildren.org/English/ages-stages/baby/feeding -nutrition/Pages/Discontinuing-the-Bottle.aspx.

266 *such as dental decay*: "Policy on Early Childhood Caries (ECC): Consequences and Preventive Strategies," in *The Reference Manual of Pediatric Dentistry* (American Academy of Pediatric Dentistry, 2024), 89–92, https://www.aapd.org/globalassets/media/policies _guidelines/p_eccconsequences.pdf.

266 *iron deficiency*: Trenna L. Sutcliffe et al, "Iron Depletion Is Associated with Daytime Bottle-Feeding in the Second and Third Years of Life," *Archives of Pediatrics & Adolescent Medicine* 160, no. 11 (2006): 1,114–20, https://doi.org/10.1001/archpedi.160.11.1114.

266 *a risk factor for obesity*: Karen Bonuck et al., "Is Overweight at 12 months Associated with Differences in Eating Behaviour or Dietary Intake Among Children Selected for Inappropriate Bottle Use?" *Maternal & Child Nutrition* 10, no. 2 (2013): 234–44, https://doi .org/10.1111/mcn.12042.

267 *Dilute the milk*: "Bottle Weaning," Texas WIC, February 25, 2025, accessed February 27, 2025, https://texaswic.org/health-nutrition /baby/bottle-weaning.

272 *whether to eat and how much*: Ellyn Satter, "Ellyn Satter's Division of Responsibility in Feeding," Ellyn Satter Institute, 2015, accessed February 6, 2025, https://www.ellynsatterinstitute.org/wp-content /uploads/2015/08/ELLYN-SATTER%E2%80%99S-DIVISION -OF-RESPONSIBILITY-IN-FEEDING.pdf.

Index

About the Author

Mallory Whitmore is a mom of two, educator, advocate, and author. She's the founder of The Formula Mom, an online platform that helps new parents make informed, confident, and supported infant-feeding decisions—without guilt or shame! When she's not working, she can be found picking up after her kids, joking with her handsome husband, reading and writing rom-coms (under the pen name Mallory Thomas), and planning trips to the beach.